CW00370308

The Effective Management of
Chronic Obstructive Pulmonary Disease

The Effective Management of Chronic Obstructive Pulmonary Disease

Edited by

Jadwiga Wedzicha MA MD FRCP

Professor of Respiratory Medicine, St Bartholomew's and the Royal London School of Medicine, St Bartholomew's Hospital, London, UK

Philip Ind MA FRCP

Senior Lecturer in Respiratory Medicine, Imperial College School of Medicine, Hammersmith Hospital, London, UK

Andrew Miles MSc MPhil PhD

Professor of Public Health Policy and UK Key Advances Series Organiser, University of East London, UK

UeL University Centre for
Public Health Policy &
Health Services Research

British
Thoracic
Society

AESCULAPIUS MEDICAL PRESS
LONDON SAN FRANCISCO SYDNEY

Published by

Aesculapius Medical Press (London, San Francisco, Sydney)
Centre for Public Health Policy and Health Services Research
Faculty of Science and Health
University of East London
33 Shore Road, London E9 7TA, UK

© Aesculapius Medical Press 2001

First published 2001

All rights reserved. No part of this publication may be reproduced or transmitted in any
form or by any means, electronically or mechanically, including photocopying, recording
or any other information storage or retrieval system, without prior permission in writing
from the publishers.

British Library Cataloguing in Publication Data
A catalogue record for this book is available from the British Library

ISBN 1 903044 19 7

While the advice and information in this book are believed to be true and accurate at the
time of going to press, neither the authors nor the publishers nor the sponsoring institutions
can accept any legal responsibility or liability for any errors or omissions that may be made.
In particular (but without limiting the generality of the preceding disclaimer) every effort
has been made to check drug usages; however, it is possible that errors have been missed.
Furthermore, dosage schedules are constantly being revised and new side-effects recognised.
For these reasons, the reader is strongly urged to consult the drug companies' printed
instructions before administering any of the drugs recommended in this book.

Further copies of this volume are available from:

Claudio Melchiorri
Research Dissemination Fellow
Centre for Public Health Policy and Health Services Research
Faculty of Science and Health
University of East London
33 Shore Road, London E9 7TA, UK

Fax: 020 8525 8661
email: claudio@keyadvances4.demon.co.uk

Typeset, printed and bound in Britain
Peter Powell Origination and Print Ltd

Contents

Contributors

Neil C Barnes MB FRCP, Consultant Respiratory Physician, London Chest Hospital, Barts and the London NHS Trust, London

David Bellamy MBE BSC DRCOG MRCGP FRCP, General Practitioner, James Fisher Medical Centre, Bournemouth

Christine E Bucknall MD MRCGP FRCP(Glas), Consultant Respiratory Physician, Hairmyres Hospital, Glasgow & Chairman, Audit Subcommittee of the British Thoracic Society, London

P Sherwood Burge MSC MD FFOM FRCP, Consultant Chest Physician, Birmingham Heartlands Hospital, Birmingham

Peter Calverley MD FRCP FRCPE, Professor of Pulmonary and Rehabilitation Medicine, Department of Medicine, University Hospital Aintree, Liverpool

John H Dark FRCS FRCP, Professor of Cardiothoracic Surgery and Consultant Cardiothoracic Surgeon, University of Newcastle and the Freeman Hospital, Newcastle-upon-Tyne

Carol L Davis FRCP, Macmillan Consultant in Palliative Medicine, Countess Mountbatten House, Moorgreen Hospital, Southampton

Elizabeth E Gamble MB MRCP, Specialist Registrar in Respiratory Medicine, London Chest Hospital, Barts and the London NHS Trust, London

Philip W Ind MA FRCP, Senior Lecturer in Respiratory Medicine, Imperial College School of Medicine at the Hammersmith Hospital, London

David A Lomas PhD FRCP, Professor of Respiratory Biology and Honorary Consultant Physician, Wellcome Trust Centre for Molecular Mechanisms in Disease, Cambridge Institute for Medical Research, University of Cambridge at Addenbrooke's Hospital, Cambridge

Philip S Marino BSC FRCP, Research Fellow in Respiratory Medicine, National Heart and Lung Institute, London

Michael DL Morgan MD MRCP, Consultant Chest Physician, Department of Respiratory Medicine and Thoracic Surgery, Glenfield Hospital, Leicester

Bippen D Patel MRCP, Clinical Research Fellow, Respiratory Medicine Unit, Department of Medicine, University of Cambridge

Mike G Pearson MB FRCP, Consultant Chest Physician, University Hospital Aintree, Liverpool and Director, Clinical Effectiveness and Evaluation Unit of The Royal College of Physicians of London

C Mike Roberts MD FRCP, Consultant Physician, Chest Unit, Whipps Cross University Hospital, London

Terence AR Seemungal MBBS MSc MRCP, British Lung Foundation Fellow, Academic Department of Respiratory Medicine, St Bartholomew's Hospital, London

Michael C Steiner, MRCP, Research Fellow, Department of Respiratory Medicine and Thoracic Surgery, Glenfield Hospital, Leicester

Nicola Stevenson MRCP, Clinical Research Fellow, Department of Medicine, University Hospital Aintree, Liverpool

Robert A Stockley MD DSC FRCP Professor of Medicine, Department of Medicine, University of Birmingham at Queen Elizabeth Hospital, Birmingham

Jadwiga A Wedzicha MA MD FRCP, Professor of Respiratory Medicine, St Bartholomew's and the Royal London School of Medicine, St Bartholomew's Hospital, London

Preface

Chronic obstructive pulmonary disease (COPD) is a major cause of mortality and morbidity which affected 44 million people in the world in 1990, and it is estimated that some 2.88 million individuals died from this condition in the year 2000. The major environmental risk factor for the development of COPD is cigarette smoking, but other environmental factors have been implicated in the development of chronic irreversible airflow obstruction. Indeed, there are associations with environmental and domestic pollution, occupational dust exposure and previous history of viral infection, and genetic factors have now been identified that can predispose a smoker to the development and progression of COPD. In primary care, COPD is significantly under-diagnosed and under-treated although, since the publication of the British Thoracic Society (BTS) guidelines for management of COPD in 1997, there has been an encouraging increase in the use of spirometry and a more systematic approach to the identification of patients in special clinics. Currently, it is believed that 1–2 per cent of an average general practice patient population will be diagnosed as showing definitive signs of the disease, although the real number of patients affected by this condition and who remain undiagnosed is probably at least twice this figure. Diagnosis therefore remains of pivotal importance to the proper management of this condition. Part 1 of this text is therefore concerned to discuss genetic predisposition and susceptibility to disease, the identification of the individual at risk and the methods through which diagnostic accuracy can be achieved and maintained.

Despite the definition of COPD as a condition associated with limited reversibility of airflow obstruction, inhaled bronchodilators remain the mainstay of drug therapy with conventional inhaled short-acting β_2 agonists being the most widely employed agents in the management of the disease. Inhaled anticholinergics have traditionally been thought to be more effective than short-acting β agonists in COPD as opposed to asthma and current thinking includes arguments that favour a combined approach. Inhaled long-acting β_2 agonists are now employed in COPD but oral β_2 agonists are little used. Slow-release theophylline preparations retain a place in treating COPD despite intolerance, potential drug interactions and their inherent toxicity, which usually requires monitoring of blood levels.

Oral corticosteroids have been widely used in the long-term management of COPD, but in general their toxicity has been considered to outweigh their benefits. Benefit has not been shown for those with very mild disease and the main uncertainties relate to the dose required and the optimal stage of disease, when the benefits of treatment begin to outweigh adverse reactions. The limitations and toxicities of existing therapies indicate the need to move towards the development of new agents and, if a drug could be convincingly shown to improve symptoms, slow the decline in lung function and therefore decrease mortality or prevent exacerbations, it would be an important new drug, providing that it could be shown to be safe.

However, because of the heterogeneous nature of the underlying pathology in COPD, it may be that new drugs will prove beneficial only in given subsets of patients. It must also be recognised, of course, that drugs that prevent weight loss or effectively treat the depression associated with COPD also have an important place in overall management.

Exacerbations of COPD are a major cause of morbidity and mortality and hospital admission, with some patients being particularly susceptible to the development of frequent exacerbations – in some cases in excess of three exacerbations per year, and these particular patients are likely to require inpatient hospital care. Respiratory viral infections represent a major cause of COPD exacerbations and the presence of an upper respiratory tract infection leads to a longer recovery time from symptoms. Other factors, including ambient temperature and interaction with environmental pollutants, may also play a role and, worryingly, in some cases lung function and symptoms fail to return to baseline levels, suggesting that exacerbations may have permanent effects on the decline of lung function. Part 2 has therefore been concerned to review the evidence and opinion for the medical management of COPD and its exacerbations, and to explore some of the common controversies that surround the definitions of optimal treatment.

Surgical intervention has, in addition to a primarily medical management, an important place in the long-term management of COPD and two surgical approaches are available for the patient with severe illness. Both have shown improvements in quality of life, but it has been difficult to demonstrate an overall survival advantage for either. Nevertheless, quality of life, as well as quantity of life, are important factors in considering management strategies in advanced disease and Part 3 reviews the evidence underpinning lung volume reduction surgery and lung transplantation. As pathological damage to the airways in COPD cannot be reversed by conventional medical and surgical intervention, rehabilitation strategies have been developed, which have aimed to reduce symptoms, reduce disability and handicap, and improve functional independence through multi-professional approaches involving programmes of physical training, disease education, nutritional, psychological, social and behavioural interventions. Part 4 reviews the British Thoracic Society statement on the management of pulmonary rehabilitation, with the aim of offering some pragmatic guidance for those colleagues who are concerned with developing such a dedicated service for local populations.

Part 5, the concluding part, sets the previous reviews of evidence and opinion within the context of service delivery as a whole and with reference to the modern policy requirements of the NHS; it incorporates a thorough review of the availability and reliability of current clinical practice guidelines for COPD management, and the organisation and delivery of effective palliative care services. In the modern policy environment, no approach to clinical management would be complete without the institution of systems for the review of clinical decision-making and its outcomes and the detection of suboptimal care or, indeed, frank error. The concluding two chapters of this final part therefore review systems of audit of COPD services, and review and classify common medical errors.

In the current age, where doctors and health professionals are increasingly overwhelmed by clinical information, we have aimed to provide a fully current, fully referenced text which is as succinct as possible but as comprehensive as necessary. Consultants in respiratory medicine and their trainees and general practitioners and their trainees are likely to find it of particular use as part of continuing professional development and specialist training, respectively, and we advance it specifically as an excellent tool for these purposes. We anticipate, however, that the volume will also prove of substantial use to nurse specialists and to all those members of the multi-disciplinary clinical team routinely involved in the management of the patient with COPD, and indeed to all those colleagues who have an interest in or direct responsibility for the provision of effective, efficient services for the investigation and management of this disabling disease.

In conclusion we thank Boehringer-Ingelheim Ltd for the grant of educational sponsorship, which helped organise a national symposium held with the British Thoracic Society at The Royal College of Physicians of London, at which synopses of the constituent chapters of this book were presented.

Jadwiga Wedzicha MA MD FRCP
Philip Ind MA FRCP
Andrew Miles MSc MPhil PhD

PART 1

Genetics, screening and diagnosis

Genetic predisposition and susceptibility to chronic obstructive pulmonary disease

Bippen D Patel and David A Lomas

Introduction

Chronic obstructive pulmonary disease (COPD) is defined as airflow obstruction that does not change appreciably over a period of several months (British Thoracic Society 1997). It is a major cause of global morbidity and mortality that affected 44 million people in 1990. Indeed, 14 million people suffer from COPD in the United States alone, where this condition resulted in nearly 92,000 deaths in 1995 (Wise 1997). It is estimated that 2.88 million people in the world will die from COPD this year (Murray & Lopez 1999) and the numbers are growing. COPD is becoming more prevalent among Western women and is set to explode in developing countries such as India, Mexico, Cuba, Egypt, South Africa and China (Peto *et al.* 1999). The environmental and genetic factors that predispose to COPD are reviewed in this chapter.

Environmental factors that predispose to COPD

The major environmental risk factor for the development of COPD is cigarette smoking. In non-smokers the forced expiratory volume in 1 second (FEV_1) declines at a mean rate of approximately 20–30 ml per year during adult life. In most smokers this mean rate of decline is increased to 30–45 ml per year but in the subset of cigarette smokers who are susceptible to developing COPD the rate of decline is 80–100 ml per year. There is evidence of a dose–response between the severity of lung disease and the pack-years of cigarettes smoked (Burrows *et al.* 1977; Fletcher & Peto 1977; Dockery *et al.* 1988; Peat *et al.* 1989) but the correlation coefficient is low indicating that only 15 per cent of the variability in FEV_1 is accounted for by this factor.

Other environmental factors have also been implicated in the development of chronic irreversible airflow obstruction. There has been a recognised association with environmental pollution since the great London smogs (Holland & Reid 1965). Domestic and cooking fumes are also important and in certain cities in China the non-smoker emphysema death rates are almost 100 times greater than those of the non-smoker in the USA (Peto *et al.* 1999). Exposure to dust in the coal and gold mining industries have both been linked to airflow obstruction (Kauffmann *et al.* 1979; Oxman *et al.* 1993) and the inhalation of dust and gases by underground tunnel workers has similarly been associated with an accelerated decline in FEV_1, respiratory symptoms and COPD when compared to matched controls who worked above ground (Ulvestad *et al.* 2000). COPD is more common in individuals of lower socio-economic status (Kauffmann *et al.* 1979) and has a poorer prognosis when associated with low body mass index (Landbo *et al.* 1999) and with bronchial hyper-reactivity (Rijcken *et al.* 1995; Eden *et al.* 1997). There is also evidence that previous viral infections predispose smokers to COPD (Matsuse *et al.* 1992) and an increasing awareness that diet (Sargeant *et al.* 2000) and factors involved during *in utero* (Barker & Osmond 1986; Barker *et al.* 1991) and adolescent lung development (Tager *et al.* 1988) may be important in the predisposition to obstructive lung disease. These factors all have an additive effect with cigarette smoking.

Alpha$_1$-antitrypsin deficiency

The only genetic risk factor that has been proven to predispose smokers to COPD is α_1-antitrypsin deficiency. α_1-Antitrypsin deficiency was first described as a clinical entity in 1963 by Laurell and Eriksson (1963) who noted an absence of the α_1 band on serum protein electrophoresis. The major function of α_1-antitrypsin is to protect the tissues against the enzyme neutrophil elastase (Beatty *et al.* 1980; Carrell *et al.* 1982). Its role in protecting the lungs against proteolytic attack is underscored by the association of plasma deficiency with early onset panlobular emphysema (Eriksson 1965), asthma (Colp *et al.* 1993), bronchiectasis (King *et al.* 1996) and Wegener's granulomatosis (Griffith *et al.* 1996). Over 70 naturally occurring variants have been described and characterised by their migration on isoelectric focusing gels (Brantly *et al.* 1988). The two most common deficiency variants, S and Z, result from point mutations in the α_1-antitrypsin gene (Jeppsson 1976; Owen *et al.* 1976; Yoshida *et al.* 1976) and make the protein migrate more slowly than normal M α_1-antitrypsin. S α_1-antitrypsin (^{264}Glu→Val) is found in up to 28 per cent of southern Europeans and, although it results in plasma α_1-antitrypsin levels that are 60 per cent of the M allele, it is not associated with any pulmonary sequelae. The Z variant (^{342}Glu→Lys) results in a more severe deficiency which is characterised, in the homozygote, by plasma α_1-antitrypsin levels of 10–15 per cent of the normal M allele. The Z mutation results in the accumulation of α_1-antitrypsin as inclusions in the rough endoplasmic reticulum of the liver. These inclusions predispose the homozygote to juvenile hepatitis, cirrhosis (Sveger 1976, 1988) and hepatocellular carcinoma (Eriksson *et al.* 1986).

The mechanism underlying α_1-antitrypsin deficiency was determined in 1992 by Lomas *et al.* The S and Z mutations destabilise the protein to allow the formation of chains of polymers which tangle within hepatocytes (Elliott *et al.* 1996b; Mahadeva *et al.* 1999). These polymers are formed by a well-defined protein–protein interaction between the reactive centre loop of one α_1-antitrypsin molecule and β-sheet A of a second (Elliott *et al.* 1996a; Sivasothy *et al.* 2000). The dimer is then able to extend to form chains of polymers which have an ordered structure and are therefore not detected by the endoplasmic reticulum surveillance system within the cell which recognises misfolded proteins (Graham *et al.* 1990).

Homozygous Z α_1-antitrypsin deficiency makes up only 1–2 per cent of all cases of COPD and there is considerable variability in FEV_1 between current and ex-smokers with the same PI Z genotype (Silverman *et al.* 1989). This suggests that other coexisting genetic factors must predispose to lung disease in Z α_1-antitrypsin homozygotes. A logical follow-on from the association of α_1-antitrypsin deficiency with emphysema is an assessment of the risk of COPD in heterozygotes who carry an abnormal Z allele and a normal M allele. These individuals have plasma α_1-antitrypsin levels that are approximately 65 per cent of normal (50 per cent from the M allele and 15 per cent from the Z allele). A population-based study demonstrated that PI MZ heterozygotes do not have a clearly increased risk of lung damage (Bruce *et al.* 1984). However, if groups of patients are collected who already have COPD, then the prevalence of PI MZ individuals appears to be elevated (Lieberman *et al.* 1986). In addition, several longitudinal studies have demonstrated that, among COPD patients, the PI MZ heterozygotes have a more rapid decline in lung function (Tarján *et al.* 1994; Sandford *et al.* 2001). These data suggest that either all PI MZ individuals are at slightly increased risk for the development of COPD, or that a subset of the PI MZ subjects are at substantially increased risk of pulmonary damage if they smoke.

Risk of COPD in individuals without α_1-antitrypsin deficiency

Several previous studies have suggested that genetic factors other than α_1-antitrypsin deficiency may be involved in the susceptibility of cigarette smokers to develop chronic airflow obstruction. These studies have demonstrated a significantly higher prevalence of COPD among relatives of index patients than among control groups (Larson *et al.* 1970; Kueppers *et al.* 1977; Rybicki *et al.* 1990). The findings have been confirmed recently in a study of 44 patients with severe COPD (FEV_1<40 per cent predicted) aged 52 or less (Silverman *et al.* 1998). The prevalence of airflow obstruction in smoking siblings was approximately threefold greater than in smoking control subjects.

Chronic obstructive pulmonary disease is a syndrome that includes chronic obstructive bronchitis, chronic irreversible asthma and emphysema. In advanced disease it is difficult to dissect out the relative contribution of each of these to airflow obstruction. The clearest phenotype of the three is emphysema which is characterised by airflow obstruction, hyperinflation, reduced diffusing capacity on lung function tests, areas of low attenuation on high-resolution CT scans and characteristic histology. Over the past three years the authors have undertaken a study to assess familial clustering of emphysema in the East Anglian region of the UK. One hundred and fifty-two patients were approached who met the criteria for severe emphysema at a relatively young age (the probands). One hundred and fifty agreed to take part in the study of whom 149 were Caucasian. The study revealed a wide range of smoking history in the probands with three individuals developing severe emphysema after having smoked only one pack of cigarettes/day for four years. The siblings and parents of each of these probands were then contacted and screened for airflow obstruction and emphysema with questionnaires and lung function tests. One hundred and seventy-nine of the 221 siblings were enrolled into the study. Detailed analysis revealed that 34 per cent of siblings who were current or ex-smokers had airflow obstruction, with a significant proportion of these also fulfilling the reduced gas transfer criteria for emphysema. A case control study is currently underway and has recruited 20 age/sex/smoking/geography matched controls. The prevalence of airflow obstruction in the unrelated matched control group is significantly lower than that in the siblings. Thus our data suggest that the emphysema component of COPD also clusters in families in the absence of α_1-antitrypsin deficiency.

Association studies

The clustering of COPD in families has resulted in the recognition of a genetic component to this multifactorial disease. There are now increasing numbers of association studies assessing genes that may predispose smokers to COPD (Table 1.1). These studies rely on two populations matched for all factors that are known to affect FEV_1 (age, sex, smoking history, occupational exposure to dusts, α_1-antitrypsin deficiency, ethnicity and bronchial hyperreactivity) but one group have irreversible airflow obstruction and the other group are unaffected. Such studies are often complicated by small numbers of patients and the difficulty in matching for all known environmental and genetic factors that predispose to COPD. It is made more difficult as some of these factors have yet to be determined. Moreover researchers can only assess genes that have already been described where they think it is biologically plausible that mutations in the protein may be associated with COPD. This candidate gene approach is relatively straightforward but the results are often difficult to interpret (Todd 1999).

The first studies using candidate genes in COPD assessed polymorphisms in the proteins that protect the lungs against proteolytic attack. A polymorphism was described in the 3'-non-coding region of α_1-antitrypsin that predisposed smokers to developing COPD (Kalsheker *et al.* 1987). This observation was confirmed by a second European group (Poller *et al.* 1990) but refuted by others (Sandford *et al.* 1997; Mahadeva *et al.* 1998; Benetazzo *et al.* 1999). Mutations resulting in partial deficiency of α_1-antichymotrypsin have similarly been associated with COPD (Poller *et al.* 1992, 1993) although they are uncommon and unlikely to play a major role in the pathogenesis of more typical disease. The cytokine tumour necrosis factor-α plays an important role in the inflammatory response, and polymorphisms that affect synthesis have been linked with COPD in smokers (Huang *et al.* 1997; Kucukaycan *et al.* 2000). Once again these findings have been refuted by others who have also assessed the association between these polymorphisms and airflow obstruction in Caucasian populations (Higham *et al.* 2000; Kucukaycan *et al.* 2000; Patuzzo *et al.* 2000).

Table 1.1 Candidate genes that have been associated with COPD in case–control studies

PI MZ α_1-antitrypsin deficiency
Tumour necrosis factor-α_1
Microsomal epoxide hydrolase
Glutathione S1-transferase
Haem oxygenase-1
Taq-1 polymorphism of α_1-antitrypsin
α_1-Antichymotrypsin
Vitamin D-binding protein
ABO blood group
ABH secretor status
Cystic fibrosis transmembrane regulator
HLA
Cytochrome P450

Each puff of a cigarette contains 10^{17} free radicals that can cause lung damage. Thus defects in the detoxification of these reactive oxygen species may predispose smokers to airflow obstruction and emphysema. Indeed the proportion of patients with slow microsomal epoxide hydrolase activity was significantly higher in patients with COPD and emphysema when compared to healthy blood donor controls (Smith *et al.* 1997). These findings have been supported by colleagues (Sandford *et al.* 2001) but refuted by others who assessed Korean (Yim *et al.* 2000) and North American (Kueppers 2000) populations. More recently, Yamada *et al.* (2000) reported an association between a short tandem repeat polymorphism in the heme oxygenase-1 gene promoter and COPD. This protein also plays an important antioxidant role in the lung, and there is in vitro evidence that the polymorphism in the promoter region reduces the upregulation of haem oxygenase-1 in response to reactive oxygen species in cigarette smoke. Finally mutations in glutathione S1-transferases that generate protective antioxidants have also been associated with the development of COPD (Ishii *et al.* 1999; Miravitlles *et al.* 2000).

The results from the association studies are confusing but taken together they suggest that there is support for the well-established hypotheses of proteinase–antiproteinase and oxidant–antioxidant imbalance causing lung damage and COPD.

Genomic scans to identify genes that predispose smokers to COPD

The association studies described above have all been conducted with variants in known candidate genes. Clearly our understanding of COPD would be revolutionised if a new gene or genes could be discovered that explained the predisposition of a minority of smokers to develop COPD. An alternative approach to this problem is to detect novel genes using linkage analysis in families of COPD patients with polymorphic markers throughout the genome. If a marker segregates with COPD in affected relatives, then it indicates that this marker is located close to a gene or genes that cause this disease. In order for this approach to be successful, it requires a large number of well-characterised affected relatives: either extended pedigrees or nuclear families can be used.

The magnitude and organisation of a network to recruit the thousands of patients that are required for such studies is extremely expensive. A pharmaceutical company (Glaxo-Wellcome) has funded a consortium that spans ten centres in seven North American and European countries. The consortium is a collaboration between universities and industry designed to recruit nuclear families of COPD patients. This consortium has started to recruit 3,000 families in order to identify 1,500 affected sib-pairs with COPD. The index cases (probands) and their siblings are being screened with respiratory questionnaires, spirometry and high-resolution chest CT scans. The collection of this data from 3,000 patients with COPD and their siblings will provide unique insights into the pathophysiology of airflow obstruction and, most importantly, the genetics of this condition.

The identification of novel genes would allow the assessment of new mechanisms and pathways in disease and provide new therapeutic opportunities. At-risk individuals could be identified by screening and strongly advised to abstain from smoking and avoid occupations where there are high loads of environmental dusts. Finally, new genes may help to explain other diseases. There is epidemiological evidence that COPD and lung cancer share a common familial component other than smoking (Cohen et al. 1977; Tockman et al. 1987). The discovery of novel genes that predispose to COPD may therefore have a major impact on our understanding of the pathogenesis of cancer.

Conclusion

Chronic obstructive pulmonary disease is a common cause of morbidity and mortality. There is increasing recognition that genetic factors, other than α_1-antitrypsin deficiency, predispose a subset of smokers to develop airflow obstruction. Several candidate genes have been proposed but the data is often controversial. It is hoped that genome wide scans on large numbers of affected sib-pairs will identify novel COPD susceptibility genes. Such a finding would revolutionise our understanding of the pathogenesis of COPD and may provide new therapeutic targets.

References

Barker DJP & Osmond C (1986). Childhood respiratory infection and adult chronic bronchitis in England and Wales. *British Medical Journal* **293**, 1271–1275

Barker DJP, Godfrey KM, Fall C, Osmond C, Winter PD, Shaheen SO (1991). Relation of birth weight and childhood respiratory infection to adult lung function and death from chronic obstructive airways disease. *British Medical Journal* **303**, 671–674

Beatty K, Bieth J, Travis J (1980). Kinetics of association of serine proteinases with native and oxidized α-1-proteinase inhibitor and α-1-antichymotrypsin. *Journal of Biological Chemistry* **255**, 3931–3934

Benetazzo MG, Gile LS, Bombieri C *et al.* (1999). α_1-Antitrypsin TAQ I polymorphism and α_1-antichymotrypsin mutations in patients with obstructive pulmonary disease. *Respiratory Medicine* **93**, 648–654

Brantly M, Nukiwa T, Crystal RG (1988). Molecular basis of alpha-1-antitrypsin deficiency. *American Journal of Medicine* **84**, 13–31

British Thoracic Society (1997). BTS guidelines for the management of chronic obstructive pulmonary disease. *Thorax* **52,** Supplement 5

Bruce RM, Cohen BH, Diamond EL *et al.* (1984). Collaborative study to assess risk of lung disease in Pi MZ phenotype subjects. *American Review of Respiratory Diseases* **130**, 386–390

Burrows B, Knudson RJ, Cline MG, Lebowitz MD (1977). Quantitative relationships between cigarette smoking and ventilatory function. *American Review of Respiratory Diseases* **115**, 195–205

Carrell RW, Jeppsson J-O, Laurell C-B *et al.* (1982). Structure and variation of human α_1-antitrypsin. *Nature* **298**, 329–334

Cohen BH, Diamond EL, Graves CG et al. (1977). A common familial component in lung cancer and chronic obstructive pulmonary disease. *Lancet* **ii**, 523–526

Colp C, Pappas J, Moran D, Lieberman J (1993). Variants of α_1–antitrypsin in Puerto Rican children with asthma. *Chest* **103**, 812–815

Dockery DW, Speizer FE, Ferris BG Jr, Ware JH, Louis TA, Spiro III A (1988). Cumulative and reversible effects of lifetime smoking on simple tests of lung function in adults. *American Review of Respiratory Diseases* **137**, 286–292

Eden E, Mitchell DBM, Khouli H, Nejat M, Grieco MH, Turino GM (1997). Atopy, asthma, and emphysema in patients with severe alpha-1-antitrypsin deficiency. *American Journal of Respiratory Critical Care Medicine* **156**, 68–74

Elliott PR, Lomas DA, Carrell RW, Abrahams J-P (1996a). Inhibitory conformation of the reactive loop of α_1-antitrypsin. *Nature Structural and Biology* **3**, 676–681

Elliott PR, Stein PE, Bilton D, Carrell RW, Lomas DA (1996b). Structural explanation for the dysfunction of S α_1-antitrypsin. *Nature Strucures Biology* **3**, 910–911

Eriksson S (1965). Studies in α_1-antitrypsin deficiency. *Acta Medica Scandinavia* **432**, 1–85

Eriksson S, Carlson J, Velez R (1986). Risk of cirrhosis and primary liver cancer in alpha$_1$-antitrypsin deficiency. *New England Journal of Medicine* **314**, 736–739

Fletcher C & Peto R (1977). The natural history of chronic airflow obstruction. *British Medical Journal* **1**, 1645–1648

Graham KS, Le A, Sifers RN (1990). Accumulation of the insoluble PiZ variant of human α_1-antitrypsin within the hepatic endoplasmic reticulum does not elevate the steady-state level of grp78/BiP. *Journal of Biological Chemistry* **265**, 20463–20468

Griffith ME, Lovegrove JU, Gaskin G, Whitehouse DB, & Pusey CD (1996). C-antineutrophil cytoplasmic antibody positivity in vasculitis patients is associated with the Z allele of alpha-1-antitrypsin, and P-antineutrophil cytoplasmic antibody positivity with the S allele. *Nephrology, Dialysis and Transplantation* **11**, 438–443

Higham MA, Pride NB, Alikhan A, Morrell NW (2000). Tumour necrosis factor-α gene promoter polymorphism in chronic obstructive pulmonary disease. *European Respiratory Journal* **15**, 281–284

Holland WW & Reid DD (1965). The urban factor in chronic bronchitis. *Lancet* **i**, 445–448

Huang S-L, Su C-H, Chang S-C (1997). Tumor necrosis factor-α gene polymorphism in chronic bronchitis. *American Journal of Respiratory and Critical Care Medicine* **156**, 1436–1439

Ishii T, Matsuse T, Teramoto S *et al.* (1999). Glutathione S-transferase P1 (GSTP1). polymorphism in patients with chronic obstructive pulmonary disease. *Thorax* **54**, 693–696

Jeppsson J-O (1976). Amino acid substitution Glu → Lys in α_1-antitrypsin PiZ. *FEBS Letters* **65**, 195–197

Kalsheker NA, Hodgson IJ, Watkins GL, White JP, Morrison HM, Stockley RA (1987). Deoxyribonucleic acid (DNA). polymorphism of the α_1-antitrypsin gene in chronic lung disease. *British Medical Journal* **294**, 1511–1514

Kauffmann F, Drouet D, Lellouch J, Brille D (1979). Twelve year spirometric changes among Paris area workers. *International Journal of Epidemiology* **8**, 201–212

King MA, Stone JA, Diaz PT, Mueller CF, Becker WJ, Gadek JE (1996). α_1-antitrypsin deficiency: evaluation of bronchiectasis with CT. *Radiology* **199**, 137–141

Kucukaycan M, van Krugten M, Pennings HJ *et al.* (2000). Tumor necrosis factor-alpha polymorphism in chronic obstructive pulmonary disease: difference in +489 genotype frequency compared with controls. *American Journal of Respiratory and Critical Care Medicine* **161**, A811

Kueppers F (2000). Predisposing factors to COPD. *American Journal of Respiratory and Critical Care Medicine* **161**, A814

Kueppers F, Miller RD, Gordon H, Hepper NG, Offord K (1977). Familial prevalence of chronic obstructive pulmonary disease in a matched pair study. *American Journal of Medicine* **63**, 336–342

Landbo C, Prescott E, Lange P, Vestbo J, Almdal TP (1999). Prognostic value of nutritional status in chronic obstructive pulmoanry disease. *American Journal of Respiratory and Critical Care Medicine* **160**, 1856–1861

Larson RK, Barman ML, Kueppers F, Fudenberg HH (1970). Genetic and environmental determinants of chronic obstructive pulmonary disease. *Annals of Internal Medicine* **72**, 627–632

Laurell C-B & Eriksson S (1963). The electrophoretic α_1-globulin pattern of serum in α_1-antitrypsin deficiency. *Scandinavian Journal of Clinical and Laboratory Investigations* **15**, 132–140

Lieberman J, Winter B, Sastre A (1986). Alpha$_1$-antitrypsin Pi-types in 965 COPD patients. *Chest* **89**, 370–373

Lomas DA, Evans DL, Finch JT, Carrell RW (1992). The mechanism of Z α_1-antitrypsin accumulation in the liver. *Nature* **357**, 605–607

Mahadeva R, Chang W-SW, Dafforn T *et al.* (1999). Heteropolymerisation of S, I and Z α_1-antitrypsin and liver cirrhosis. *Journal of Clinical Investigation* **103**, 999–1006

Mahadeva R, Westerbeek R, Perry DJ *et al.* (1998). α_1-Antitrypsin deficiency alleles and the Taq-1 G→A allele in cystic fibrosis lung disease. *European Respiratory Journal* **11**, 873–879

Matsuse T, Hayashi S, Kuwano K, Keunecke H, Jefferies WA, Hogg JC (1992). Latent adenoviral infection in the pathogenesis of chronic airways obstruction, *American Review of Respiratory Diseases* **146**, 177–184

Miravitlles M, Jardi R, Gonzalez C *et al.* (2000). Genetic polymorphism of glutathione S-tranferase P1 gene and chronic obstructive pulmonary disease. *American Journal of Respiratory and Critical Care Medicine* **161**, A208

Murray CJL & Lopez AD (1999). *Global Burden of Disease and Injury Series,* volume II: *Global Health Statistics: A compendium of incidence, prevalence, and mortality estimates for over 200 conditions.* Harvard School of Public Medicine

Owen MC, Carrell RW, Brennan SO (1976). The abnormality of the S variant of human α_1-antitrypsin. *Biochimica Biophysica Acta* **453**, 257–261

Oxman AD, Muir DCF, Shannon HS, Stock SR, Hnizdo E, Lange HJ (1993). Occupational dust exposure and chronic obstructive pulmonary disease. A systematic overview of the evidence. *American Review of Respiratory Diseases* **148**, 38–48

Patuzzo C, Gile LS, Zorzetto M *et al.* (2000). Tumor necrosis factor gene complex in COPD and disseminated bronchiectasis. *Chest* **117**, 1353–1358

Peat JK, Woolcock AJ, Cullen K (1989). Decline of lung function and development of chronic airflow limitation: a longitudinal study of non-smokers and smokers in Busselton, Western Australia. *Thorax* **45**, 32–37

Peto R, Chen Z-M, Boreham J (1999). Tobacco-the growing epidemic. *Nature Medicine* **5**, 15–17

Poller W, Faber J-P, Scholz S *et al.* (1992). Mis-sense mutation of α_1-antichymotrypsin gene associated with chronic lung disease. *Lancet* **339**, 1538

Poller W, Faber J-P, Weidinger S *et al.* (1993). A leucine-to-proline substitution causes a defective α_1-antichymotrypsin allele associated with familial obstructive lung disease. *Genomics* **17**, 740–743

Poller W, Meisen C, Olek K (1990). DNA polymorphisms of the α_1-antitrypsin gene region in patients with chronic obstructive pulmonary disease. *European Journal of Clinical Investigations* **20**, 1–7

Rijcken B, Schouten JP, Xu X, Rosner B, Weiss ST (1995). Airway hyperresponsiveness to histamine associated with accelerated decline in FEV_1. *American Journal of Respiratory and Critical Care Medicine* **151**, 1377–1382

Rybicki BA, Beaty TH, Cohen BH (1990). Major genetic mechanisms in pulmonary function. *Journal of Clinical Epidemiology* **43**, 667–675

Sandford AJ, Spinelli JJ, Weir TD, Paré PD (1997). Mutation in the 3' region of the α-1-antitrypsin gene and chronic obstructive pulmonary disease. *Journal of Medicine and Genetics* **34**, 874–875

Sandford AJ, Chagani T, Weir TD *et al.* (2001). Susceptibility genes for rapid decline of lung function in the lung health study. *American Journal of Respiratory and Critical Care Medicine* **163**, 469–473

Sargeant LA, Jaeckel A, Wareham NJ (2000). Interaction of vitamin C on the relation between smoking and obstructive airways disease in EPIC-Norfolk. *European Respiratory Journal* **3**, 397–403

Silverman EK, Chapman HA, Drazen JM *et al.* (1998). Genetic epidemiology of severe, early-onset chronic obstructive pulmonary disease. *American Journal of Respiratory and Critical Care Medicine* **157**, 1770–1778

Silverman EK, Province MA, Campbell EJ, Pierce JA, Rao DC (1989). Biochemical intermediates in α_1-antitrypsin deficiency: residual family resemblance for total α_1-antitrypsin, oxidised α_1-antitrypsin, and immunoglobulin E after adjustment for the effect of the Pi locus. *Genetic Epidemiology* **7**, 137–149

Sivasothy P, Dafforn TR, Gettins PGW, Lomas DA (2000). Pathogenic $\alpha_1$antitrypsin polymers are formed by reactive loop-β-sheet A linkage. *Journal of Biological Chemistry* **275**, 33663–33668

Smith CAD & Harrison DJ (1997). Association between polymorphism in gene for microsomal epoxide hydrolase and susceptibility to emphysema. *Lancet* **350**, 630–633

Sveger T (1976). Liver disease in alpha$_1$-antitrypsin deficiency detected by screening of 200,000 infants. *New England Journal of Medicine* **294**, 1316–1321

Sveger T (1988). The natural history of liver disease in α_1-antitrypsin deficient children. *Acta Paediatrica Scandinavica* **77**, 847–851

Tager IB, Segal MR, Speizer FE, Weiss ST (1988). The natural history of forced expiratory volumes. Effect of cigarette smoking and respiratory symptoms. *American Reviews in Respiratory and Critical Care Medicine* **138**, 837–849

Tarján E, Magyar P, Váczi Z, Lantos Å, Vaszár L (1994). Longitudinal lung function study in heterozygous PiMZ phenotype subjects. *European Respiratory Journal* **7**, 2199–2204

Tockman MS, Anthonisen NR, Wright EC, Donithan MG (1987). Airways obstruction and the risk for lung cancer. *Annals of Internal Medicine* **106**, 512–518

Todd JA (1999). Interpretation of results from genetic studies of multifactorial diseases. *Lancet* **354**, s15–s16

Ulvestad B, Bakke B, Melbostad E, Fuglerud P, Kongerud J, Lund MB (2000). Increased risk of obstructive pulmonary disease in tunnel workers. *Thorax* **55**, 277–282

Wise RA (1997). Changing smoking patterns and mortality from chronic obstructive pulmoanry disease. *Preventative Medicine* **26**, 418–421

Yamada N, Yamaya M, Okinaga S *et al.* (2000). Microsatellite polymorphism in the heme oxygenase-1 gene promoter is associated with susceptibility to emphysema. *American Journal of Human Genetics* **66**, 187–195

Yim J-J, Park GY, Lee C-T *et al.* (2000). Genetic susceptibility to chronic obstructive pulmonary disease in Koreans: combined analysis of polymorphic genotypes for microsomal epoxide hydrolase and glutathione S-transferase M1 and T1. *Thorax* **55**, 121–125

Yoshida A, Lieberman J, Gaidulis L, Ewing C (1976). Molecular abnormality of human alpha$_1$–antitrypsin variant (Pi-ZZ). associated with plasma activity deficiency. *Proceedings of the National Academy of Sciences of the USA* **73**, 1324–1328

Chapter 2

Identification of the individual at risk, the utility of opportunistic screening in the primary healthcare setting and the place of spirometry

David Bellamy

Introduction

Chronic obstructive pulmonary disease (COPD) is a common and clinically important disease complex in primary care affecting at least 1 per cent of the total practice population. It is significantly under-diagnosed and less than half the sufferers are correctly identified. Diagnosis of the early stages of the disease is made more difficult as patients are likely to be relatively free of symptoms until lung function has fallen to 60 per cent or less of the normal value. Symptoms are usually first noticed after the age of 50 and many smokers will not be surprised to have developed a morning productive 'smokers' cough or mild breathlessness on exertion correctly attributable to their long history of smoking. As a result they usually fail to consult a doctor about their perceived problems. Even when seen at a surgery consultation, they are unlikely to mention mild symptoms unless specifically asked.

It is well recognised that the only intervention that will prevent progression of COPD is to stop smoking. If the disease is to be stopped before the development of symptoms, a new strategy will need to be developed in primary care which will include such measures as screening smokers over 40 with spirometry to look for early evidence of airflow obstruction. There will also need to be a major education campaign for smokers to alert them of the symptoms of COPD, and encourage them to see GPs and practice nurses to discuss the symptoms and appropriate management with help and advice to stop smoking. Such campaigns are currently being developed by the British Thoracic Society (BTS) COPD Consortium and the British Lung Foundation with the aid of posters that will be widely displayed in surgeries and public places.

Raising the profile of COPD in primary and secondary care and at governmental level should help health workers to give COPD the time and appropriate management it commands. COPD has been largely neglected in the last 30 years but with the publication of the BTS Guidelines in 1997 interest has been stimulated in primary care and needs much input and nurturing to diagnose and manage this disease effectively.

What is the extent of the problem?

COPD causes considerable morbidity and a poor quality of life for many patients with more severe levels of airflow obstruction. Until recently, the disorder has been largely neglected in primary care with advice usually being limited to telling patients that they must stop smoking and that little else could be done for them. COPD constitutes a large workload for general practice with more consultations and more hospital admissions than asthma. On average, patients with COPD have two to three acute exacerbations per year and therapy costs per patient far exceed those of asthma, largely due to the high cost of oxygen therapy.

In an average primary care group (PCG) which comprises about 100,000 patients there will be:

- 1,000 diagnosed cases of COPD
- 238 admissions (of asthma 178)
- 55 deaths per year
- 25 per cent of deaths occurring before retirement age
- GP consultations costing £43,649 per year
- drug therapy costing £781 per patient per year (asthma £198).

Identifying patients

Practices are beginning to set up procedures to identify, diagnose and more effectively manage COPD. As with asthma, a team approach is often employed with trained practice nurses playing a key role in the assessment, performing spirometry and patient follow-up. A varied approach will be adopted depending on the level of interest, expertise and staff available. The patient groups which may be evaluated might include the following, the later ones being studied with increasing experience and time commitment:

- those with an existing diagnosis of chronic bronchitis and emphysema;
- patients over 40 labelled as asthmatic or taking bronchodilators who also smoke;
- smokers who have symptoms of breathlessness, cough, sputum, wheeze or acute exacerbations of bronchitis;
- asymptomatic smokers over 40;
- patients who may self-refer in response to posters displayed in surgeries;
- patients referred by pharmacists who see them about coughs.

Practices are being increasingly encouraged to record clinical data on computer databases so that audit of clinical practice may be performed. An example of the clinical data that could readily be recorded might be:

– smoking history
– MRC dyspnoea grade
– spirometry FEV$_1$ (per cent predicted)
  mild/moderate/severe
– bronchodilator reversibility

– steroid reversibility
– oxygen saturation
– home nebuliser
– home oxygen
– pneumococcal vaccine given

Such data will also provide invaluable information on the pattern of COPD in the community.

Figure 2.1 shows the distribution of COPD severity by percentage FEV$_1$ in the first 85 patients who have been evaluated in the author's practice.

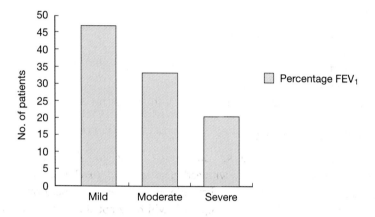

Figure 2.1 Distribution of COPD severity by percentage FEV$_1$ in 85 patients

The role of spirometry in primary care

Perhaps the greatest challenge in COPD management is to encourage a more widespread, accurate and appropriate use of spirometry in the community.

Until the publication of the BTS COPD Guidelines in 1997, COPD management had been largely neglected and was very much considered a disease process for which little could or, indeed, needed to be done other than to suggest patients gave up smoking. The use of spirometers on a regular basis to diagnose and assess severity of COPD was minimal.

In 1996, a postal survey of 2,548 randomly selected general practitioners in the UK revealed that of the 931 who returned the questionnaire 39 per cent had a spirometer in their practice (Bellamy *et al.* 1997). Of those who owned or were intending to buy a spirometer, 86 per cent said that the practice nurse would carry out the testing. Ninety per cent agreed the nurse needed appropriate training. At the time of the survey, 61 per cent of the owned spirometers were of the simple hand-held electronic variety with no graphical display. Disappointingly, only 11 per cent of responders had access to local open access spirometry at the local hospital. The disadvantage of postal surveys is that the data obtained tends to be biased by the interests of those who return the questionnaire. It is therefore likely that the true figures for the proportion of practices with a spirometer was considerably less than 39 per cent.

When the BTS COPD Guidelines were produced, a considerable effort was put into disseminating an attractively presented four-page summary to a wide range of health professionals. All primary care physicians received a copy as well as approximately 15,000 practice nurses who were known to have an interest in asthma or who ran clinics in asthma. This mailing, coupled with postgraduate meetings and the setting up of training courses in COPD and spirometry for practice nurses, greatly increased the awareness of COPD, its effective treatment, and the measurement of FEV_1 to make a diagnosis and assessment of disease severity.

Primary care practitioners are now systematically evaluating patients with chronic respiratory symptoms, many of whom have been diagnostically labelled as asthmatic, to determine the correct diagnosis and assess severity and reversibility. The most appropriate therapy can then be provided. An analysis of 100 consecutive patients with respiratory symptoms referred for spirometry in a large general practice in Kent by Pinnock *et al.* (1999) has clearly outlined the value of spirometry. Sixty five patients with airflow obstruction were identified and with bronchodilator reversibility testing, COPD differentiated from asthma. Twelve previously unsuspected restrictive defects were diagnosed, with the remainder being normal.

In the last three years many practices have purchased spirometers, a high proportion of which have the preferred facility for graphical display and thus allow more effective evaluation of blowing technique and reproducibility. Hospital pulmonary function laboratories are also making access for lung function testing more readily available.

A face-to-face marketing survey of 209 GPs and 102 practice nurses carried out on behalf of the BTS COPD Consortium by Rudolf in 1999 revealed that 50 per cent of GPs and 69 per cent of practice nurses had spirometers in their practices. Where there was no spirometer in the practice, over 75 per cent sent patients to the local hospital for lung function testing. Spirometers are used in primary care twice as often by nurses than by GPs. Encouragingly 93 per cent of the nurses had received some training in spirometry against 60 per cent of GPs. The survey is to be repeated after the circulation of a simple, practical booklet covering the uses, technique and interpretation of spirometry in primary care, first published in September 2000.

Spirometric screening of asymptomatic smokers

Since some degree of impaired lung function is likely to be measurable by the age of 40–50 years in the 20 per cent of smokers who are susceptible to tobacco smoke, there might appear to be some logic in screening this group of smokers to detect early disease. Symptomatic COPD may be totally prevented if patients can be persuaded to quit smoking at this early stage of mild airflow obstruction.

As attractive an idea as this may initially seem, there are many questions that need to be asked about the efficacy, manpower implications and cost–benefits of widespread screening before it can become routine practice in primary care. There is little in the way of data on the prevalence of mild airflow obstruction in asymptomatic smokers aged over 40 years. A study in general practice by Freeman (2000) found 19 smokers with mild or moderate levels of COPD in the first 100 patients she screened.

Likewise, there have been no studies to measure the effect on smoking quit rates if smokers are found to have abnormal lung function. It is always difficult to persuade symptomatic COPD suffers to stop smoking but will the knowledge that their lungs are not normal encourage a greater proportion to quit smoking? This would surely be a primary goal of screening. A large controlled study is urgently needed.

A negative aspect of spirometric screening of smokers might be a reassurance that, if their lung function is normal, then it is perfectly alright to continue smoking.

Large-scale screening in primary care will have considerable time and cost implications, particularly for practice nurse involvement. Screening could be opportunistic or more formalised into special clinics. However, formal evaluation needs to take account of the cost–benefit ratio of such screening.

How can quality control of measurement be achieved in primary care?

Whereas respiratory technicians in hospital have at least one year's formal training in respiratory function testing, no such schemes exist in primary care. Training of practice nurses at best may run to one- to two-day courses, some of which will deal with affiliated topics other than pure spirometry. Courses for GPs are likely to be no more than a half-day session which may provide the basics but contains little in-depth knowledge.

Hospital technicians will check and calibrate equipment daily but, depending on the type of spirometer, no such regular calibration is likely to occur in primary care. If spirometry occurs in designated clinics equipment can be calibrated beforehand, but, since much work in primary care is opportunistic and appointments are likely to be less than ten minutes in duration, there is often no time. There is thus an attraction for GPs to purchase electronic spirometers where manufacturers say no calibration is required except on annual services. Being able to switch on a spirometer and type in height, age and sex details and immediately be able to perform the blows is much more compatible with the hectic pace of a general practice surgery. The accuracy, linearity and reproducibility of electronic spirometers have recently been reviewed by a Dutch group (Schermer *et al.* 2000). They suggest good correlation between electronic spirometers and conventional spirometers. Reproducibility of FEV_1 and

FVC over time appears to be quite acceptable. The choice of spirometer for primary care should certainly be influenced by the way it is likely to be used. Opportunistic measurements definitely require a very quick and simple to use machine. Clinics can better utilise machines where more calibration has to be performed initially.

Whichever spirometer is selected it is essential that the doctor or nurse is fully aware of patient preparation, the technique for performing the blows, the problems that arise with poor blows and the criteria for good reproducibility. Knowledge is also needed to interpret traces and figures.

Quality assurance

The limited published literature on quality assurance of spirometry in primary care paints a rather gloomy picture. A recent study from New Zealand (Eaton *et al.* 1999) assessed the effect of a training workshop for doctors and practice nurses where particular attention was paid to the practical aspects of spirometry and quality assurance. Over the following 12 weeks, 'trained' staff and a control group who did not attend the spirometry workshop performed tasks on an electronic hand-held Vitalograph device that had the capability of alerting operators when the quality of blows was poor, e.g., a slow start, and also gave the level of variance between blows. All blows were analysed for acceptability on the fairly strict ATS criteria. Only 18.9 per cent of the 'trained' group and 5.1 per cent of the 'controls' performed three acceptable blows. Two acceptable blows (which may be adequate for primary care) were achieved in 33.1 per cent of 'trained' and 12.5 per cent of control groups. The main reason for non-acceptability was largely ascribed to failure to satisfy a blow lasting at least six seconds. The study suggests that the majority of FEV_1 measurements may thus be acceptable.

The study also demonstrated a good learning effect from the workshop. However, in a random selection of 559 traces, only 55 per cent were shown to have the correct interpretation when reviewed by expert pulmonologists.

A study from the Netherlands (Den Otter *et al.* 1997) examined the quality of instruction and subsequent patient use of the spirometer in a group of practice nurses or practice assistants who had been given several training sessions. Overall, about half the instructors and half the patient performance items were considered to be carried out satisfactorily. One of the main criticisms was that nurses did not bully patients sufficiently to make them produce a maximal exhalation!

Conclusions

Interest and enthusiasm in the assessment and management of COPD has been kindled, particularly in practice nurses. This will hopefully lead to a more holistic approach to the many needs of sufferers of this common and disabling disease, providing a worthwhile improvement in quality of life to patients and greater satisfaction to health professionals.

Spirometry is obviously in its infancy as a diagnostic tool in primary care. To establish reliable, accurate and reproducible spirometric readings together with the knowledge to interpret traces correctly, there needs to be: a large number of quality, accredited teaching courses; follow-up assessment of practical and theoretical knowledge; encouragement for primary care to become involved in performing spirometry; and support and teaching from local respiratory physicians and lung function laboratory staff.

It is unrealistic to assume that, in the near future, primary care will achieve the high standards of accuracy demanded from an accredited hospital respiratory function unit. Primary care must be encouraged and nurtured to start performing spirometry. The essential training process involved must always emphasise quality and correct technique.

The types of spirometers used in primary care will need to be simple to use and access, provide real-time graphical displays and printouts and be fairly inexpensive. Most will be electronic devices which have the added advantage of being small, portable and containing technology that will allow storing of multiple blows and provide instant feedback on reproducibility of blows. They also calculate predicted values thus saving the busy practitioner valuable time. By hospital standards such equipment may be thought inferior and possibly inaccurate, particularly where calibration is not regularly performed. However, they definitely fulfil the role and clinical needs of primary care in helping to screen, diagnose and assess severity of COPD as well as giving valuable information about many other forms of respiratory disease.

References

Bellamy D, Hoskins G, Smith B *et al.* (1997). The use of spirometers in general practice. *Asthma in General Practice* **5**, 8–9

British Thoracic Society (1997). Guidelines for the management of chronic obstructive pulmonary disease. *Thorax* **52**, S1–28

Den Otter JJ, Knitel M, Akkermans RPM *et al.* (1997). Spirometry in general practice: the performance of practice assistants scored by lung function technicians. *British Journal of General Practice* **47**, 41–42

Eaton T, Withy S, Garrett JE *et al.* (1999). Spirometry in primary care practice. The importance of quality assurance and the impact of spirometry workshops. *Chest* **116**, 416–423

Freeman D (2000). COPD prevalence in asymptomatic smokers – the first 100. *Asthma in General Practice* **9**(suppl 23), A48

Pinnock H, Carley-Smith J, Kalideen D (1999). Spirometry in primary care: An analysis of the first 100 patients referred in one general practice. *Asthma in General Practice* **7**, 23–24

Rudolf M (1999). Making spirometry happen. *Thorax* **54**, A43

Schermer TRJ, Folgering HTM, Bottema BJAM *et al.* (2000). The value of spirometry for primary care: asthma and COPD. *Primary Care Respiratory Journal* **9**, 51–55

Chapter 3

The importance of achieving diagnostic accuracy

Robert A Stockley

Introduction

Chronic obstructive pulmonary disease (COPD) is a disease syndrome, which presents a major challenge for healthcare workers and healthcare resources. By the year 2020 COPD is predicted to become the fifth leading cause of morbidity and mortality worldwide (Murray & Lopez 1996). It is this awareness of the healthcare burden of COPD that has resulted in rapidly expanding interest in its nature, effects and current and future managements.

The major strategies that are being undertaken include early detection and the institution of appropriate preventative measures, the continued development and application of guidelines, and the development of new therapeutic strategies based on modulation of the pathogenic processes involved.

Although COPD has now become the universal term used to describe this important clinical syndrome, in the past, clinical and pathological terms, such as chronic bronchitis and emphysema have also been used as well as other more generic terms, including chronic obstructive lung disease (COLD) and chronic obstructive airways disease (COAD). It has, however, long been recognised that these generic terms include a variety of conditions. The best recognised Venn diagram (Figure 3.1)

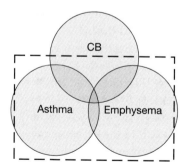

Figure 3.1 This is a Venn diagram of the interrelationship between chronic bronchitis (CB), asthma and emphysema. The dotted box delineates patients with evidence of airflow obstruction. Note that many patients with chronic bronchitis do not have airflow obstruction whereas a small proportion of patients with emphysema, as seen on high-resolution CT scan, may have no airflow obstruction in the early stages

includes three overlapping aspects namely bronchitis, emphysema and asthma. By general acceptance the patient has to have largely irreversible airflow obstruction and conventionally a diagnosis of bronchiectasis has excluded patients from this grouping. Nevertheless, if we are to apply clinical guidelines and develop new therapeutic strategies it is critical that we should ensure that our patient phenotype is well described. For instance, large multicentre studies of therapies following myocardial infarct show advantages to a variety of drugs including beta blockers, ACE inhibitors and the 'statins'. Guidelines now suggest that all such therapies should be given to patients post-myocardial infarct with some differences depending on the type of infarct. However, it remains recognised that, even in large studies, only a small proportion of the patients benefit from the therapy. The same is therefore likely to be true in COPD and with the renewed interest in this group of conditions and their management it seems appropriate to reconsider our assessment of these patients in order to identify distinct subsets that may need and respond to individual therapies.

Definition

It is generally accepted that COPD is a slowly progressive condition most notably associated with cigarette smoking (British Thoracic Society 1997), although similar pathological changes can occur in non-smokers which may of course relate to different mechanisms. Patients should have airflow obstruction that does not change markedly, although the degree of reversibility of this airflow obstruction can also vary (see below). The presence of airflow obstruction is a feature of several pathological processes and may reflect the development of emphysema (either panlobular or centrilobular), the presence of abnormalities in the small airways which may include fibrosis, narrowing of small airways due to airway wall inflammation and oedema, occlusion of the airway lumen by secretion and dynamic collapse of the airways as a result of loss of connective tissue support. In addition, bronchitis and bronchiectasis may be associated with COPD although conventionally the latter has been excluded. However, recent data have suggested that radiological evidence of bronchiectasis is often a feature of COPD in the absence of clear clinical features (see later).

It has become conventional to divide COPD patients into those with mild, moderate or severe impairment. This classification is dependent upon the measurement of the forced expiratory volume in 1 second (FEV_1). In general a value of greater than 80 per cent predicted is assumed to reflect the healthy population although recent data would suggest this may not be the case (see below). **Mild** airflow obstruction occurs in the group with an FEV_1 of 60–79 per cent predicted, **moderate** have an FEV_1 of 40–59 per cent predicted and **severe** have an FEV_1 less than 40 per cent predicted (British Thoracic Society 1997). The arbitrary definition does reflect some difference in terms of symptomatology since those with mild airflow obstruction usually have little breathlessness unless they are exceptionally athletic, those with moderate impairment have breathlessness on exertion, whereas those with severe airflow obstruction have breathlessness even on mild exertion (British Thoracic Society 1997). Similarly, it is assumed that the use of healthcare resources varies such that mild patients are pre-symptomatic, those with moderate impairment are predominantly known to primary care doctors with intermittent complaints, whereas severe impairment is found in patients likely to be known to both the primary and secondary care physicians. Again, these concepts are generalisations based on few data and may, therefore, be incorrect.

The FEV_1 as a defining measurement although relatively simple may lead to uncertainty about the diagnosis or severity. The FEV_1 is effort dependent and can also be reduced in other conditions, such as restrictive lung disease and abnormalities in the large airways. As indicated above the contribution from the small airways and the presence of dynamic airway collapse are likely to be the major factors that influence the FEV_1 in COPD. However, in these patients the forced vital capacity (FVC) can also become impaired leading to an FEV_1/FVC ratio that may be within or close to the normal range. For this reason it has become conventional now to use the vital capacity or the slow vital capacity, which minimises dynamic airways collapse during a forced manoeuvre and gives a better guide to the presence of airflow obstruction.

With this in mind a recent study (O'Brien *et al.* 2000) investigated the physiological features of a group of patients who presented to primary care with an exacerbation of presumed COPD (Figure 3.2). In this study 30 per cent of the patients

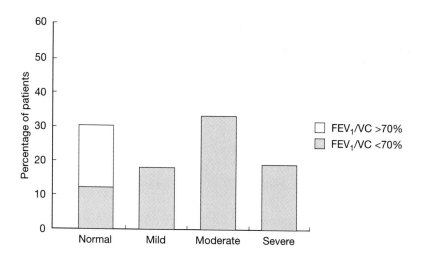

Figure 3.2 Proportion of patients presenting with an FEV_1 in the 'normal range' (greater than 80 per cent predicted): mild, moderate and severe impairment (British Thoracic Society 1997). The proportion of patients with a reduced FEV_1/FVC ratio (less that 70 per cent) is demonstrated by the hatched areas. Data obtained from O'Brien *et al.* (2000)

had an FEV_1 that was within the normal range (equal to or greater than 80 per cent predicted). In these patients 41 per cent had a reduced FEV_1/VC ratio indicating the presence of airflow obstruction. Clearly, this group is not pre-symptomatic in that they had presented to primary care and, although their FEV_1 alone suggested that they should not have airflow obstruction, comparison with the VC indicated they had. Of importance, this group could be identified with appropriate spirometry and represents the mildest form of impairment and hence patients who should be targeted for preventative therapy (smoking cessation).

Eighteen per cent of the patients with a diagnosis of COPD had mild impairment of FEV_1 in the 60–79 per cent predicted range, indicating that these patients also present with symptomatology to primary care physicians, again identifying a significant number of patients who ought to be targeted for future preventative therapy. The remaining patients with moderate and severe airflow obstruction represent patients with persistent symptoms and would be the groups targeted for effective intervention therapy.

Reversibility of airflow obstruction is conventionally tested in patients with COPD, although the general belief is that such patients have little or no reversibility of airflow obstruction when challenged acutely with bronchodilators. It is becoming increasingly recognised, however, that some patients do have a clinically important degree of reversibility. The criteria used to determine reversibility vary internationally but in the UK this is taken to be an increase in FEV_1 that is both greater than 200 ml and at least a 15 per cent increase over the pre-bronchodilator value. Using these criteria recent data (O'Brien et al. 2000) indicated that such a bronchodilator response occurred in between 40 and 55 per cent of patients whether classified as having mild, moderate or severe airflow obstruction. Furthermore, it is also recognised that patients can have a significant improvement in vital capacity and/or air trapping following bronchodilator therapy even if the FEV_1 changes little. This can be reflected by a clear increase in patients' health status. Whether the site of airflow obstruction and the presence or absence of reversibility indicate separate pathological processes remains unknown. Nevertheless, reversibility of airflow limitation at whatever site in the lung is undoubtedly related to an improvement in health status on appropriate therapy (Jones & Bosch 1997).

Trial of steroids

Many patients with COPD are treated long term with either inhaled corticosteroids or (occasionally) oral therapy and it has been conventional (where possible) to assess patients with a trial of steroid therapy. Indeed in the recent ISOLDE study a significant improvement in FEV_1 was seen during the run-in period when a course of oral steroid therapy was given (Burge et al. 2000). Such a positive trial usually results in administration of long-term therapy with inhaled corticosteroids although often such treatment is prescribed in patients with the most severe airflow obstruction even in the absence of a positive steroid trial. Steroid trials can be valuable in that a positive trial does predict a better overall improvement in lung function even though positive bronchodilator responses show individual variations, often becoming negative and vice versa (Davies *et al.* 1999b). However, once again it may be only a subset of patients that respond in such a way and these may have a pathologically different disease. Recent studies of the cell biology have indicated that patients who have a greater number of eosinophils or their products in lung secretions are more likely to respond with an increase in FEV_1 following corticosteroid therapy (Pizzichini *et al.* 1998). This clearly represents a subset of patients and may indicate those with a more asthmatic phenotype (see later). Indeed, the asthmatic component may also be relevant during exacerbations and some workers have shown that the number of eosinophils in the airway or sputum of 'COPD' patients increases during the exacerbation (Saetta *et al.* 1996). Good controlled studies have indicated that steroid therapy for exacerbations leads to a more rapid resolution of symptoms (Davies *et al.* 1999a; Niewoehner *et al.* 1999) when studied as a group. It remains uncertain whether this represents a subset response within the group since careful patient characterisation has not been undertaken.

However, studies of antibiotic therapy for exacerbations have led to some more rational selection of subsets. Controlled trials of antibiotics for acute exacerbations have often proven negative, although meta-analysis does confirm that antibiotics lead to better resolution of the episode (Saint *et al.* 1995). However, in these studies the characteristics of the exacerbations have remained poorly defined. More recently consensus opinion has indicated that an exacerbation should be defined as a persistent deterioration in symptoms beyond normal daily variability that requires intervention therapeutically (Rodriguez-Roisin 2000). Undoubtedly, some exacerbations are bacterial in origin, but determining the role of bacteria has proven difficult as patients with COPD often have bacterial colonisation even in the stable clinical state (Monso *et al.* 1995) and sputum culture may prove to be positive in 30–40 per cent of patients with chronic bronchitis and COPD. During exacerbations the positive culture rate may rise to 50 per cent (Grossman 1998), leaving a further 50 per cent with negative cultures. Clearly, the remaining 50 per cent would not be expected to require or indeed respond to antibiotic therapy, whereas the former 50 per cent may expect to show an advantage of antibiotic therapy. When the two groups are put together it could be predicted that it will be difficult to identify a positive effect for antibiotic therapy unless the numbers studied are large.

In what remains the best study of antibiotic therapy for exacerbations so far, Anthonisen *et al.* (1987) attempted to sub-classify the exacerbations depending upon the symptoms at presentation which included increased breathlessness, increased sputum volume and increased sputum purulence as major symptoms. Although patients often had minor symptoms the analysis of antibiotic response concentrated on the major symptoms alone. This controlled trial showed once again a benefit for antibiotic therapy for the exacerbations as a whole. However, subset analysis of the data presented indicated that it was only in patients who had all three major symptoms where a statistically significant benefit from antibiotic therapy was present. In retrospect this observation makes sense because sputum purulence would have to be a constant feature of the exacerbations with all three symptoms present. Sputum purulence represents a neutrophilic response (Stockley *et al.* 2000) which is the classic host defence response to bacterial infection (Stockley 1998b). Since antibiotics are known to facilitate the removal of bacteria this would be expected to be related to a resolution of neutrophilic associated inflammation and new symptoms. Indeed, in a recent study (Stockley *et al.* 2000) patients with COPD presenting with an acute exacerbation were characterised specifically into those with purulent sputum and those with mucoid sputum. The bacterial characteristics of those with mucoid sputum were similar during the exacerbation as in the stable clinical state (Figure 3.3). On the other hand, those with purulent sputum nearly always had a positive bacterial culture. Following antibiotic therapy the sputum became sterile in some 60 per cent of these patients and in those where the culture remained positive the bacterial numbers were reduced by approximately two orders of magnitude (Stockley *et al.* 2000). Again, careful subset characterisations of patients both theoretically and practically indicate a different type of process and hence choice of therapy.

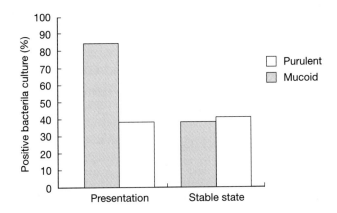

Figure 3.3 The proportion of sputum samples from patients with chronic bronchitis and an acute exacerbation of COPD is shown both at presentation and in the stable clinical state. Note that patients who present with purulent sputum have a markedly increased rate of bacterial isolation at presentation, whereas in the stable state when their secretions have returned to mucoid the incidence of bacterial isolation is similar to that seen in general COPD. Data derived from Stockley *et al.* (2000)

Other information has suggested that patients with recurrent exacerbations have the worst health status (Seemungal *et al.* 1998), indicating that these patients and this process should be targeted for future management. Studies comparing frequent and infrequent exacerbators have indicated that there may be biochemical differences that reflect or indeed lead to the differences in clinical phenotype (Bhowmik *et al.* 2000; Gompertz *et al.* 2001).

Pathogenesis

Eriksson and Laurell (1963) described five individuals identified with α_1-antitrypsin deficiency. Three of them had severe emphysema at an early age implicating the deficiency in their condition. Over the next 20 years a variety of animal experiments and some clinical studies investigated the mechanisms responsible. It was shown that enzymes from the neutrophil were capable of producing changes in both the airways and periphery of the lung that are consistent with human chronic bronchitis and emphysema (Stockley 1998a). These observations lead to the proteinase/anti-proteinase theory of the pathogenesis of emphysema with a clear belief that neutrophil elastase was the key mediator of the pathological changes and that α_1-antitrypsin was an important protective inhibitor in this respect (Stockley 1998a). In recent years this concept has been questioned; indeed there is major debate as to whether enzymes from the neutrophil are of importance in COPD rather than those from the macrophage. Studies have involved the use of bronchoalveolar lavage, bronchial lavage, spontaneous collection of sputum or the induction of sputum using hypertonic saline. These methods of harvesting secretions not only sample different areas of the bronchial tree but also different pathological processes. For instance, the spontaneous production of sputum is likely to reflect a different process to that studied by the use of induced sputum where the patients do not normally expectorate. In addition, the majority of studies being carried out in patients do not, usually, define their physiological, clinical and radiological features in detail. Thus, it is uncertain whether the patients have emphysema, loss of small airways or the occlusion/dynamic collapse of the small airways or the presence or absence of chronic bronchitis, all of which will influence the data obtained. Furthermore, even when studying airway disease, the continued habit of smoking, colonisation by bacteria, the presence or absence of eosinophils (Hill *et al.* 2000) and the presence of bronchiectasis will all influence the results obtained. With this in mind it is of interest that recent studies using high-resolution CT scanning once again differentiate subsets of patients with COPD. For instance, emphysema was visualised in approximately 50 per cent of patients with reduced FEV_1 and was even present to a limited degree in subjects with an FEV_1 greater than 80 per cent predicted (O'Brien *et al.* 2000). On the other hand, bronchiectasis was also present in approximately 30 per cent of patients, although this was of the mild tubular variety and not apparent clinically (O'Brien *et al.* 2000). Nevertheless, studies of lung secretions from these patients show the presence of a greater degree of inflammation compared to matched patients who had no bronchiectasis. These results again indicate a differential inflammatory response related to anatomical and pathological differences.

Relevance to disease management

Despite finding clear subsets of patients generically labelled as having COPD it is not certain how this influences the management of the condition. If the overall response is to administer the same medication irrespective of the patient's pathological or clinical phenotype, then clearly careful characterisation is inappropriate.Nevertheless, the widespread use of inhaled bronchodilators and/or oral corticosteroids and antibiotic therapy in particular should not be condoned. Bacterial resistance is becoming a worldwide problem and careful directed use of antibiotic therapy is mandatory. Characterising subsets of exacerbations may facilitate the more rational use of antibiotic therapy. In addition, careful monitoring of physiological responses may indicate subsets of patients who benefit more from β_2 agonists rather than anticholinergic agents. This approach will become more important as newer therapies are developed for the management of COPD based on our understanding of the pathogenesis. It is critical that we develop and direct our therapies with the pathological processes in mind. For instance, inhaled therapy may be appropriate for problems that are predominantly bronchial in origin although not if the problem lies in the alveolar region where drug penetration may be inadequate. In addition specific treatments for emphysema may not be appropriate for patients with bronchial disease or where the major cause of their ill-health and progression is recurrent infective exacerbations.

Spirometry is clearly mandatory for diagnosing the presence of airflow obstruction. However, further physiological assessment as well as determination of the symptoms and the radiological appearance of the lungs may all help in understanding individual responses, the effects of smoking, pollution and infection, and determining targeted therapy. This concept has been proposed recently by Boushey (1999) who stated: 'Different mechanism of inflammation that underlie COPD must be defined before specific therapies can be tailored to treat them.'

References

Anthonisen NR, Manfreda J, Warren CP et al. (1987) Antibiotic therapy in exacerbations of chronic obstructive pulmonary disease. *Annals of Internal Medicine* **106**, 196–204

Bhowmik A, Seemungal TAR, Sapsford RJ et al. (2000). Relationship of sputum inflammatory changes to symptoms and lung function changes in COPD exacerbations. *Thorax* **55**, 114–120

British Thoracic Society (1997). BTS guidelines for the management of chronic obstructive pulmonary disease. *Thorax* **52**, S1–S28

Boushey HA (1999). Gluco-corticoid therapy for chronic obstructive pulmonary disease. *New England Journal of Medicine* **340**, 1990–1991

Burge PS, Calverley PMA, Jones PW *et al.* (2000). Randomised double-blind placebo controlled study of fluticasone propionate in patients with moderate to severe chronic obstructive pulmonary disease: the Isolde Trials. *British Medical Journal* **320**, 1297–1303

Davies L, Angus RM, Calverley PMA (1999a). Oral corticosteroids in patients admitted to hospital with exacerbations of chronic obstructive pulmonary disease: a prospective randomised controlled trial. *Lancet* **354**, 456–460

Davies L, Nisar M, Pearson MG, Costello RW, Earis JE, Calverley PM (1999b). Oral corticosteroid trial in the management of stable chronic obstructive pulmonary disease. *Quarterly Journal of Medicine* **92**, 395–400

Eriksson S & Laurell C-B (1963). A new abnormal serum globulin α_1-antitrypsin. *Acta Chemica Scandinavica* **17**, S150–S153

Gompertz S, Baildey DL, Hill SL, Stockley RA (2001). The relationship between airway inflammation and frequency of exacerbations in patients with smoking–related COPD. *Thorax* **56**, 36–41

Grossman RF (1998). The value of antibiotics and the outcomes of antibiotic therapy in exacerbations of COPD. *Chest* **113**, 249S–255S

Hill AT, Gompertz S, Stockley RA (2000). Inflammation in COPD. *Thorax* **55**, 970–977

Jones PW & Bosch TK (1997). Quality of life changes in COPD patients treated with Salmeterol. *American Journal of Respiratory and Critical Care Medicine* **155**, 1283–1289

Monso E, Ruiz J, Rosell A *et al.* (1995). Bacterial infection on chronic obstructive pulmonary disease: a study of stable and exacerbated out-patients using the protected specimen brush. *American Journal of Respiratory and Critical Care Medicine* **152**, 1316–1320

Murray C J L & Lopez A D (1996). Evidence-based health policy: lessons from the global burden of disease study. *Science* **274**, 740–743

Niewoehner DE, Erbland ML, Deupree RH *et al.* (1999). Effect of systemic gluco-corticoids on exacerbations of chronic obstructive pulmonary disease. *New England Journal of Medicine* **340**, 1941–1947

O'Brien C, Guest PJ, Hill SL, Stockley RA (2000). Physiological and radiological characterisation of patients diagnosed with chronic obstructive pulmonary disease in primary care. *Thorax* **55**, 635–642

Pizzichini E, Pizzichini MMM, Gibson P *et al.* (1998). Sputum eosinophilia predicts benefit from Prednisone in smokers with chronic obstructive bronchitis. *American Journal of Critical Care Medicine* **158**, 1511–1517

Rodriguez-Roisin R (2000). Towards a consensus definition for COPD exacerbations. *Chest* **117**, 398S–401S

Saetta M, Di Stefano A, Maestrelli P *et al.* (1996). Airway eosinophilia and expression of interleukin –5 in asthma and in exacerbations of chronic bronchitis. *Clinical Experiments in Allergy* **26**, 766–774

Saint S, Bent S, Vittinghoff E *et al.* (1995). Antibiotics in chronic obstructive pulmonary disease exacerbations: a meta-analysis. *Journal of the American Medical Association* **273**, 957–960

Seemungal TAR, Donaldson GC, Paul EA *et al.* (1998). Effect of exacerbation on quality of life in patients with chronic obstructive pulmonary disease. *American Journal of Respiratory and Critical Care Medicine* **157**, 1418–1422

Stockley RA (1998a). Obstructive airways disease: proteases/anti-proteases: pathogenesis and role in therapy. *Clinical Pulmonary Medicine* **5**, 203–210

Stockley RA (1998b). Role of bacteria in the pathogenesis and progression of acute and chronic lung infection. *Thorax* **53**, 58–62

Stockley RA, O'Brien C, Pye A, Hill SL (2000). Relationship of sputum colour to nature and out-patient management of exacerbations of COPD. *Chest* **117**, 1638–1645

PART 2

Evidence and opinion for medical intervention

Chapter 4

Current thinking on the nature of exacerbation and the time course and recovery of exacerbations of COPD

Jadwiga A Wedzicha and Terence AR Seemungal

Introduction

Exacerbations of chronic obstructive pulmonary disease (COPD) contribute to 30,000 deaths per year in the UK and are an important cause of the considerable morbidity found in patients with COPD. Some patients are prone to frequent exacerbations that are an important cause of hospital admission and readmission, which may have considerable impact on activities of daily living and well-being (Osman *et al.* 1997; Seemungal *et al.* 1998). COPD exacerbations are associated with considerable physiological deterioration although there is no little information available on the longer-term effects of an exacerbation.

Causes of COPD exacerbations include viral and bacterial infection and exposure to common pollutants. Although exacerbations are more common in the winter months when there are more viral infections in the community, viruses have been recognised as an important factor in asthmatic exacerbations (Nicholson *et al.* 1993; Johnston *et al.* 1995), little attention has been paid to the effects of viral infection on COPD exacerbation. Viral infections are important potential therapeutic targets that could potentially reduce exacerbation, hospital admission and thus mortality.

Epidemiology of COPD exacerbation

Earlier descriptions of COPD exacerbations had concentrated mainly on studies of hospital admission, although most COPD exacerbations are treated in the community and not associated with hospital admission. The authors followed a cohort of moderate to severe COPD patients in east London (East London COPD Study – Seemungal *et al.* 1998) with daily diary cards and peak flow readings, who were asked to report exacerbations as soon as possible after symptomatic onset. The diagnosis of COPD exacerbation was based on criteria modified from those described by Anthonisen *et al.* (1987), which require two symptoms for diagnosis, one of which must be a major symptom of increased dyspnoea, sputum volume or sputum purulence. Minor exacerbation symptoms included cough, wheeze, sore throat, nasal discharge or fever. It was found that approximately 50 per cent of exacerbations were unreported to the research team, despite considerable encouragement provided, and only diagnosed from diary cards, although there were no differences in major symptoms or physiological parameters between reported and unreported exacerbations (Seemungal *et al.* 1998). Patients with COPD are accustomed to frequent symptom changes and thus may tend to under-report exacerbations to physicians. These patients have high levels of anxiety and depression and may accept their situation (Okubadejo *et al.* 1996). The tendency of patients to under-report exacerbations may explain the higher total rate of exacerbation at 2.7 per patient per year, which is higher than previously reported by Anthonisen *et al.* (1987) at 1.1 per patient per year. However, in the latter study, exacerbations were unreported and diagnosed from patients' recall of symptoms.

Using the median number of exacerbations as a cut-off point, COPD patients in the East London Study were classified as frequent and infrequent exacerbators. Quality of life scores were measured using a validated disease specific scale – the St George's Respiratory Questionnaire (SGRQ) – and were significantly worse in all components (symptoms, activities and impacts) in the frequent, compared to the infrequent, exacerbators. This suggests that exacerbation frequency is an important determinant of health status in COPD and is thus an important outcome measure in COPD. Factors predictive of frequent exacerbations included daily cough and sputum and frequent exacerbations in the previous year. A previous study of acute infective exacerbations of chronic bronchitis found that one of the factors predicting exacerbation was the number in the previous year (Ball *et al.* 1995), although this study was limited to exacerbations presenting with purulent sputum and no physiological data were available.

In a further prospective analysis of 504 exacerbations, where daily monitoring was performed, there was some deterioration in symptoms, although no peak flow changes (Seemungal *et al.* 2000a). Falls in peak flow and forced expiratory volume in 1 second (FEV_1) at exacerbation were generally small and not useful in predicting exacerbations, but larger falls in peak flow were associated with symptoms of dyspnoea, presence of colds or related to longer recovery time from exacerbations. Symptoms of dyspnoea, common colds, sore throat and cough increased significantly during the prodromal phase and this suggests that respiratory viruses have early effects on exacerbations. The median time to recovery of peak flow was six days and seven days for symptoms, but at 35 days peak flow had returned to normal in only 75 per cent of exacerbations, while at 91 days 7.1 per cent of exacerbations had not returned to baseline lung function. Recovery was longer in the presence of increased dyspnoea or symptoms of a common cold at exacerbation. The changes observed in lung function at exacerbation were smaller than those observed at asthmatic exacerbations, although the average duration of an asthmatic exacerbation was longer at 9.6 days (Reddel *et al.* 1999; Tattersfield *et al.* 1999).

As exacerbations may not fully recover to baseline states, this suggests that COPD exacerbation may lead to the progressive decline in lung function, characteristic of

COPD, although there is no evidence currently available for this hypothesis. Increased airway inflammation is associated with faster deterioration of lung function and, as airway inflammatory markers are increased in patients with frequent exacerbations, this group may show a faster decline and hence increased mortality. Further studies are required on the relationship between exacerbation and decline in physiological function. The reasons for the incomplete recovery of symptoms and lung function are not clear, but may involve inadequate treatment or persistence of the causative agent. The association of the symptoms of increased dyspnoea and of the common cold at exacerbation with a prolonged recovery suggests that viral infections may lead to more prolonged exacerbations. As colds are associated with longer exacerbations, COPD patients who develop a cold may be prone to more severe exacerbations and should be considered for therapy early at onset of symptoms.

Airway inflammation at exacerbation

Although it has been assumed that exacerbations are associated with increased airway inflammation, there has been little information available on the nature of inflammatory markers especially when studied close to an exacerbation, as performing bronchial biopsies at exacerbation is difficult in moderate to severe COPD. The relation of any airway inflammatory changes to symptoms and physiological changes at exacerbations is also an important factor to consider. In one study, where biopsies were performed at exacerbation in patients with chronic bronchitis, increased airway eosinophilia was found, although the patients studied had only mild COPD (Saetta *et al.* 1994). With exacerbation, there were more modest increases observed in neutrophils, T lymphocytes (CD3) and tumour necrosis factor α (TNF-α)-positive cells, while there were no changes in CD4 or CD8 T cells, macrophages or mast cells. However, the technique of sputum induction allows study of these patients at exacerbation and we have shown that it is a safe and well-tolerated technique in COPD patients (Bhowmik *et al.* 1998). Levels of inflammatory cytokines have been shown to be elevated in induced sputum in COPD patients when stable, although changes at exacerbation had not been previously studied (Keatings *et al.* 1996).

The authors prospectively followed a cohort of patients from the East London COPD Study and related inflammatory markers in induced sputum to symptoms and physiological parameters both at baseline and at exacerbation (Bhowmik *et al.* 2000). There was a relation between exacerbation frequency and sputum cytokines, in that there were increased sputum interleukins IL-6 and IL-8 found in patients at baseline when stable with frequent exacerbations compared to those with infrequent exacerbations, although there was no relation between cytokines and baseline lung function. Sputum cell counts were not increased at baseline in patients with more frequent exacerbations, suggesting that the increased cytokine production comes from the bronchial epithelium in COPD. As discussed below, exacerbations are triggered by viral infections, especially by rhinovirus which is the cause of the common cold.

Rhinovirus has been shown to increase cytokine production in an epithelial cell line (Subauste *et al.* 1995) and thus repeated viral infection may lead to upregulation of cytokine airway expression.

At exacerbation, the authors found increases in induced sputum IL-6 levels and the levels of IL-6 were higher when exacerbations were associated with symptoms of the common cold. Experimental rhinovirus infection has been shown to increase sputum IL-6 in normal subjects and asthmatics (Fraenkel *et al.* 1995; Grunberg *et al.* 1997; Fleming *et al.* 1999). However, rises in cell counts and IL-8 were more variable with exacerbation and did not reach statistical significance, suggesting marked heterogeneity in the degree of the inflammatory response at exacerbation. The exacerbation IL-8 levels were related to sputum neutrophil and total cell counts, indicating that neutrophil recruitment is the major source of airway IL-8 at exacerbation. Lower airway IL-8 has been shown to increase with experimental rhinovirus infection in normal and asthmatic patients in some studies (Grunberg *et al.* 1997), but not in others (Fleming *et al.* 1999). However, COPD patients already have up-regulated airway IL-8 levels when stable due to their high sputum neutrophil load (Keatings *et al.* 1996) and further increases in IL-8 would be unlikely. COPD exacerbations are associated with a less pronounced airway inflammatory response than asthmatic exacerbations (Pizzichini *et al.* 1997), and this may explain the relatively reduced response to steroids seen at exacerbation in COPD patients, relative to asthma (Albert *et al.* 1980; Thompson *et al.* 1996; Davies *et al.* 1999; Niewoehner *et al.* 1999). We have also recently shown that the mediator endothelin-1 which may be produced by airway epithelial cells is also increased in induced sputum at COPD exacerbation and this rise is related to the sputum Il-6 levels (Roland *et al.* 2001). Endothelin-1 may be produced in reponse to stimulation by IL-6 and has also been shown to be synthesised in relation to respiratory viral infection (Carr *et al.* 1998). Thus a number of different mediators may interact at exacerbation and further study of airway inflammatory change at exacerbation is required.

In contrast to previous findings, the authors did not detect an increase in eosinophil count at exacerbation, even though their patients were sampled early at exacerbation with onset of symptoms. Compared to the study by Saetta *et al.* (1994), where patients had mild COPD, the authors' patients had more severe and irreversible airflow obstruction with an FEV_1 at 39 per cent predicted. Thus it is possible that the inflammatory response at exacerbation is different in nature in patients with moderate to severe COPD than in patients with milder COPD.

As patients were followed with daily diary cards, the authors could also relate the inflammatory markers to exacerbation recovery. There was no relation between the degree of inflammatory cell response with exacerbation and duration of symptoms and lung function changes. Induced sputum markers taken 3–6 weeks after exacerbation showed no relation to exacerbation changes. Thus levels of induced sputum markers at exacerbation do not predict the subsequent course of the exacerbation and will not be useful in the prediction of exacerbation severity.

Aetiology of COPD exacerbation

COPD exacerbations have been associated with a number of aetiological factors, including infection and pollution episodes. COPD exacerbations are frequently triggered by upper respiratory tract infections and these are more common in the winter months, when there are more respiratory viral infections in the community. Patients may also be more prone to exacerbations in the winter months as lung function in COPD patients shows small but significant falls with reduction in outdoor temperature during the winter months (Donaldson *et al.* 1999). COPD patients have been found to have increased hospital admissions, suggesting increased exacerbations, when increasing environmental pollution occurs. During the December 1991 pollution episode in the UK, COPD mortality was increased together with an increase in hospital admission in elderly COPD patients (Anderson *et al.* 1995). However, common pollutants, especially oxides of nitrogen and particulates, may interact with viral infection to precipitate exacerbation rather than acting alone.

Viral infections

Viral infections are an important trigger for COPD exacerbations. Studies in childhood asthma have shown that viruses, especially rhinovirus (the cause of the common cold), can be detected by polymerase chain reaction from a large number of these exacerbations (Johnston *et al.* 1995). Rhinovirus has not hitherto been considered to be of much significance during exacerbations of COPD. In a study of 44 chronic bronchitics over two years, Stott *et al.* (1968) found rhinovirus in 13 (14.9 per cent) of 87 exacerbations of chronic bronchitis. In a more detailed study of 25 chronic bronchitics with 116 exacerbations over four years, Gump *et al.* (1976) found that only 3.4 per cent of exacerbations could be attributed to rhinoviruses. In a more recent study of 35 episodes of COPD exacerbation using serological methods and nasal samples for viral culture, little evidence was found for a rhinovirus aetiology of COPD exacerbation (Philit *et al.* 1992).

We have recently shown that up to approximately one third of COPD exacerbations were associated with viral infections, and 75 per cent of these were due to rhinovirus, when samples were taken from nasopharyngeal aspirates (Harper-Owen *et al.* 1999). Viral exacerbations were associated with symptomatic colds and prolonged recovery. However, the authors found that rhinovirus was recovered from induced sputum more frequently than from nasal aspirates at exacerbation, suggesting that wild-type rhinovirus can infect the lower airway and contribute to exacerbation inflammatory changes (Seemungal *et al.* 2000b). The authors also found that exacerbations associated with the presence of rhinovirus in induced sputum had larger increases in airway IL-6 levels. Other viruses may trigger COPD exacerbation, although coronavirus was associated with only a small proportion of asthmatic exacerbations and is unlikely to play a major role in COPD (Nicholson *et al.* 1993; Johnston *et al.* 1995).

Bacterial colonisation

Airway bacterial colonisation has been found in approximately 30 per cent of COPD patients. This figure has been shown to be related to the degree of airflow obstruction, current cigarette smoking, airway neutrophil count and airway inflammatory markers (Soler *et al.* 1999; Zalacain *et al.* 1999). Although bacteria such as *Haemophilus influenzae* and *Streptococcus pneumoniae* have been associated with COPD exacerbation, some studies have shown increasing bacterial counts during exacerbation, while others have not confirmed these findings (Monso *et al.* 1999; Wilson 1999). Patients with exacerbations associated with purulent sputum are more likely to have increased bacterial counts, compared to patients with exacerbations associated with no sputum or mucoid sputum only. There is no current evidence that patients with frequent exacerbations have increased sputum bacterial colonisation when stable to explain the higher cytokine levels observed. Cultures of bronchial epithelial cells showed increased cyoktine IL-6 production after stimulation with endotoxin (Khair *et al.* 1994). However, it is also possible that there may be interactions between viral and bacterial infection at COPD exacerbation. Other organisms such as *Chlamydia pneumoniae*, which have been associated with asthmatic exacerbation, may also play a role in COPD exacerbation. We found little evidence of *C. pneumoniae* in nasopharyngeal samples, although there was greater isolation of *C. pneumoniae* in induced sputum (Harper-Owen *et al.* 2000).

Systemic inflammatory effects of COPD exacerbations

In addition to airway inflammatory effects of COPD exacerbations, systemic inflammatory effects may also be observed at COPD exacerbations. We studied levels of the systemic inflammatory markers, plasma fibrinogen and systemic IL-6 in patients in our cohort, both when stable and at exacerbation. We found that the stable plasma fibrinogen level was raised at 3.86 g/l, compared to 3.1 g/l in a sample of normal patients of similar age (Wedzicha *et al.* 2000). Plasma fibrinogen is an independent risk factor for cardiovascular disease and this rise in stable fibrinogen increases the risk of coronary heart disease in these COPD patients by 60 per cent. Reports have suggested a relationship between COPD and increased cardiovascular mortality (Jousilahti *et al.* 1996; Haider *et al.* 1999). At exacerbation we found further rises in fibrinogen and also rises in IL-6. Multiple regression showed greater rises of fibrinogen in patients when exacerbations were associated with purulent sputum and symptomatic colds. Thus COPD exacerbations may be associated with viral and bacterial infections, which could lead to increases of airway and systemic IL-6 and thus stimulate a rise in plasma fibrinogen. This proposes a mechanism for the association between acute respiratory tract infection and coronary artery disease, through increased thrombogenicity. COPD exacerbation may be an important risk factor for morbidity and mortality from cardiovascular disease.

Conclusions

COPD exacerbations are an important cause of morbidity and this paper has described some important characteristics of COPD exacerbations. Some patients with COPD seem prone to frequent exacerbations that are one of the most important determinants of health status, and thus patients with frequent exacerbation are an important group to target with respect to preventive therapy. Patients who develop frequent exacerbations have higher levels of airway inflammatory markers when stable, suggesting that exacerbation could contribute to the progressive airway inflammation characteristic of COPD. Inflammatory responses at COPD exacerbation are variable, but rises in inflammatory markers are related to the presence of upper respiratory tract infection. Rhinoviral infection is the most important aetiological factor in COPD exacerbations and is an important target for preventive therapy. Reduction of COPD exacerbation will have an important impact on the considerable morbidity and mortality associated with COPD.

References

Albert RK, Martin TR, Lewis SW (1980). Controlled clinical trial of methylprednisolone in patients with chronic bronchitis and acute respiratory insufficiency. *Annals of Internal Medicine* **92**, 753–758

Anderson HR, Limb ES, Bland JM, Ponce de Leon A, Strachan DP, Bower JS (1995). Health effects of an air pollution episode in London, December 1991. *Thorax* **50**, 1188–1193

Anthonisen NR, Manfreda J, Warren CPW, Hershfield ES, Harding GKM, Nelson NA (1987). Antibiotic therapy in exacerbations of chronic obstructive pulmonary disease. *Annals of Internal Medicine* **106**, 196–204

Ball P, Harris JM, Lowson D, Tillotson G, Wilson R (1995). Acute infective exacerbations of chronic bronchitis. *Quarterly Journal of Medicine* **88**, 61–68

Bhowmik A, Seemungal TAR, Sapsford RJ, Devalia JL, Wedzicha JA (1998). Comparison of spontaneous and induced sputum for investigation of airway inflammation in chronic obstructive pulmonary disease. *Thorax* **53**, 953–956

Bhowmik A, Seemungal TAR, Sapsford RJ, Wedzicha JA (2000). Relation of sputum inflammatory markers to symptoms and physiological changes at COPD exacerbations *Thorax* **55**, 114–200

Carr MJ, Spalding LJ, Goldie RG *et al.* (1998). Distribution of immunoreactive endothelin in the lungs of mice during respiratory viral infection. *European Respiratory Journal* **11**, 79–85

Davies L, Angus RM, Calverley PMA (1999). Oral corticosteroids in patients admitted to hospital with exacerbations of chronnic obstructive pulmonary disease, a prospective randomised controlled trial. *Lancet* **354**, 456–460

Donaldson GC, Seemungal T, Jeffries DJ, Wedzicha JA (1999). Effect of environmental temperature on symptoms, lung function and mortality in COPD patients. *European Respiratory Journal* **13**, 844–849

Fleming HE, Little EF, Schnurr D *et al.* (1999). Rhinovirus-16 colds in healthy and asthmatic subjects. *American Journal of Respiratory and Critical Care Medicine* **160**, 100–108

Fraenkel DJ, Bardin PG, Sanderson G *et al.* (1995). Lower airways inflammation during rhinovirus colds in normal and in asthmatic subjects. *American Journal of Respiratory and Critical Care Medicine* **151**, 879–886

Grunberg K, Smits HH, Timmers MC *et al.* (1997). Experimental rhinovirus 16 infection, effects on cell differentials and soluble markers in sputum of asthmatic subjects. *American Journal of Respiratory and Critical Care Medicine* **156**, 609–616

Gump DW, Phillips CA, Forsyth BR (1976). Role of infection in chronic bronchitis. *American Review of Respiratory Diseases* **113**, 465–473

Haider AW, Larson MG, O'Donnell CJ *et al.* (1999). The association of chronic cough with the risk of myocardial infarction, the Framingham Heart Study. *American Journal of Medicine* **106**, 279–284

Harper-Owen R, Seemungal TAR, Bhowmik A, Johnston SL, Jeffries DJ, Wedzicha JA (1999). Virus and Chlamydia isolation in COPD exacerbations. *European Respiratory Journal* **14**, 47s

Harper-Owen R, Seemungal TAR, Johnston SL, Jeffries DJ, Wedzicha JA (2000). Role of *Chlamydia pneumoniae* in COPD exacerbations. *American Journal of Respiratory and Critical Care Medicine* **3**, 807

Johnston SL, Pattemore PK, Sanderson G *et al.* (1995). Community study of the role of viral infections in exacerbations of asthma in 9-11 year old children. *British Medical Journal* **310**, 1225–1229

Jousilahti P, Vartiainen E, Tuomilehto J, Puska P (1996). Symptoms of chronic bronchitis and the risk of coronary disease. *Lancet* **348**, 567–572

Keatings VM, Collins PD, Scott DM *et al.* (1996). Differences in Interleukin-8 and Tumour Necrosis Factor in induced sputum from patients with chronic obstructive pulmonary disease and asthma. *American Journal of Respiratory and Critical Care Medicine* **153**, 530–534

Khair OA, Devalia JL, Abdelaziz MM, Sapsford RJ, Tarraf H, Davies RJ (1994). Effect of *Haemophilus influenzae* endotoxin on the synthesis of IL-6, IL-8, TNF-α and expression of ICAM1 in cultured human bronchial epithelial cells. *European Respiratory Journal* **7**, 2109–2116

Monso E, Rosell A, Bonet G *et al.* (1999). Risk factors for lower airway bacterial colonization in chronic bronchitis. *European Respiratory Journal* **13**, 338–342

Nicholson KG, Kent J, Ireland DC (1993). Respiratory viruses and exacerbations of asthma in adults. *British Medical Journal* **307**, 982–986

Niewoehner DE, Erbland ML, Deupree RH *et al.* (1999). Effect of systemic glucocorticoids on exacerbations of chronic obstuctive pulmonary disease. *New England Journal of Medicine* **340**, 1941–1947

Okubadejo AA, Jones PW, Wedzicha JA (1996). Quality of life in patients with chronic obstructive pulmonary disease and severe hypoxaemia. *Thorax* **51**, 44–47

Osman LM, Godden DJ, Friend JAR, Legge JS, Douglas JG (1997). Quality of life and hospital re-admission in patients with chronic obstructive pulmonary disease. *Thorax* **52**, 67–71

Philit F, Etienne J, Calvet A *et al.* (1992). Infectious agents associated with exacerbations of chronic obstructive pulmonary disease and attacks of asthma. *Rev Mal Respir* **9**, 191–196

Pizzichini MMM, Pizzichini E, Clelland *et al.* (1997). Sputum in severe exacerbations of asthma, kinetics of inflammatory indices after prednisone treatment. *American Journal of Respiratory and Critical Care Medicine* **155**, 1501–1508

Reddel HS, Ware S, Marks G, Salome C, Jenkins C, Woolcock A (1999). Differences between asthma exacerbations and poor asthma control. *Lancet* **353**, 364–369

Roland MA, Bhowmik A, Sapsford RJ *et al.* (2001). Sputum and plasma endothelin-1 at exacerbation of chronic obstructive pulmonary disease. *Thorax* in press

Saetta M, Di Stefano A, Maestrelli P *et al.* (1994). Airway eosinophilia in chronic bronchitis during exacerbations. *American Journal of Respiratory and Critical Care Medicine* **150**, 1646–1652

Seemungal TAR, Donaldson GC, Paul EA , Bestall JC, Jeffries DJ, Wedzicha JA (1998). Effect of exacerbation on quality of life in patients with chronic obstructive pulmonary disease. *American Journal of Respiratory and Critical Care Medicine* **157**, 1418–1422

Seemungal TAR, Donaldson GC, Bhowmik A, Jeffries DJ, Wedzicha JA (2000a). Time course and recovery of exacerbations in patients with chronic obstructive pulmonary disease. *American Journal of Respiratory and Critical Care Medicine* **161**, 1608–1613

Seemungal TAR, Harper-Owen R, Bhowmik A, Jeffries DJ, Wedzicha JA (2000b). Detection of rhinovirus in induced sputum at exacerbation of chronic obstructive pulmonary disease. *European Respiratory Journal* **16**, 677–683

Soler N, Ewig S, Torres A, Filella X, Gonzalez J, Zaubet A (1999). Airway inflammation and bronchial microbial patterns in patienst with stable chronic obstructive pulmonary disease. *European Respiratory Journal* **14**, 1015–1022

Stott EJ, Grist NR, Eadie MB (1968). Rhinovirus infections in chronic bronchitis, isolation of eight possible new rhinovirus serotypes. *Journal of Medical Microbiology* **109**, 117

Subauste MC, Jacoby DB, Richards SM, Proud D (1995). Infection of a human respiratory epithelial cell line with rhinoovirus. *Journal of Clinical Investigations* **96**, 549–557

Tattersfield AE, Postma DS, Barnes PJ *et al.* (1999). Exacerbations of asthma. *American Journal of Respiratory and Critical Care Medicine* **160**, 594–599

Thompson WH, Nielson CP, Carvalho P *et al.* (1996). Controlled trial of oral prednisolone in outpatients with acute COPD exacerbation. *American Journal of Respiratory and Critical Care Medicine* **154**, 407–412

Wedzicha JA, Seemungal TAR, MacCallum PK *et al.* (2000). Acute exacerbations of chronic obstructive pulmonary disease are accompanied by elevations of plasma fibrinogen and serum IL-6 levels. *Thrombosis and Haemostasis* **84**, 210–215

Wilson R (1999). Bacterial infection and chronic obstructive pulmonary disease. *European Respiratory Journal* **13**, 233–235

Zalacain R, Sobradillo V, Amilibia J *et al.* (1999). Predisposing factors to bacterial colonization in chronic obstructive pulmonary disease. *European Respiratory Journal* **13**, 343–348

Chapter 5

Scientific evidence and expert clinical opinion for the selection and use of bronchodilators: clinical decision making in the individual patient

Philip S Marino and Philip W Ind

Introduction

Despite the definition of chronic obstructive pulmonary disease (COPD) as a condition associated with limited reversibility of airflow obstruction, inhaled bronchodilators remain the mainstay of drug therapy. This chapter will focus on the use of bronchodilators in clinical assessment and clinical trial data regarding treatment of patients with COPD, excluding the management of acute exacerbations of disease. Inhaled and oral bronchodilators in routine use are listed in Table 5.1.

Table 5.1 Bronchodilator therapy for treatment of COPD

Inhaled	Short-acting β_2 agonists	Salbutamol Terbutaline Fenoterol Reproterol	Multiple inhaler devices Aerosol
	Long-acting β_2 agonists	Salmeterol Eformoterol	CFC-free dry powder
	Anticholinergics	Ipratropium Oxitropium	Nebuliser solutions, etc.
	Combined preparations	Combivent Duovent	available
Oral	Short-acting β_2 agonists	Salbutamol Terbutaline	
	Slow-release β_2 agonists	Salbutamol Terbutaline	Sustained- release preps
	Long-acting β_2 agonists	Bambuterol	Prodrug
	Methylxanthines	Theophylline Aminophylline	Multiple slow- release preps

Physiological considerations

Bronchodilator drugs act to increase airway calibre and relieve obstruction to airflow. This occurs predominantly by relaxation of smooth muscle tone in peripheral and central airways, but other mechanisms may be involved. The effect achieved will depend on the particular drug, the dose administered, the concentration arriving at the relevant receptors, baseline tone, disease inhomogeneity and, importantly, the test used to measure change. Bronchodilatation may be demonstrated by improvement in any test of airway functional although forced expiratory volume in 1 second (FEV_1), peak expiratory flow (PEF) and, in some countries, plethysmography are used most. Reduction of dynamic hyperinflation may occur with improved lung emptying, reduced functional residual capacity (FRC) and work of breathing. In addition to direct effects on airway smooth muscle, bronchodilators, particularly β_2 agonists, may exert effects on various other cell types (Table 5.2).

Inhaled β_2-adrenoceptor agonists

Conventional, inhaled, short-acting β_2 agonists are the most widely used bronchodilators. They produce rapid-onset, short-lasting, limited relief of symptoms, particularly breathlessness. They are well tolerated and no clinically significant effects of tolerance have been described in COPD.

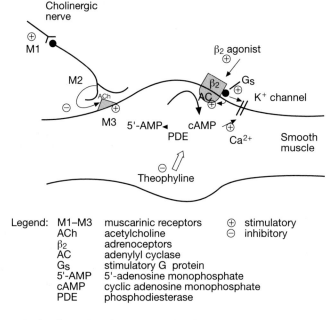

Legend:
M1–M3	muscarinic receptors	⊕	stimulatory
ACh	acetylcholine	⊖	inhibitory
β2	adrenoceptors		
AC	adenylyl cyclase		
Gs	stimulatory G protein		
5'-AMP	5'-adenosine monophosphate		
cAMP	cyclic adenosine monophosphate		
PDE	phosphodiesterase		

Figure 5.1 Mechanism of action of bronchodilators

Mechanism of action

β_2 Agonists produce all their effects by activation of cell surface β_2 receptors (Figure 5.1). The most important are situated on airway smooth muscle, although they are widely distributed. β_1 Receptors are of little importance in the lung (Table 5.2). β_2-Receptor stimulation increases intracellular cyclic adenosine monophosphate (cAMP) through a stimulatory coupling G protein (G_s) activating protein kinase A (PKA), which phosphorylates a number of intracellular proteins. PKA directly inhibits myosin light chain kinase and also phosphoinositol hydrolysis, reducing intracellular calcium concentrations. This stimulates a variety of processes leading to smooth muscle relaxation. It is also clear, however, that a direct effect, mediated via G_s, leading to opening of membrane potassium channels, may be important at low β_2 agonist concentrations.

Table 5.2 Lung β_2 and muscarinic receptors: site and potential pharmacological effects

	Type	Agonist Action	Effect	Result
β_2-Adrenoceptors				
Airway smooth muscle:				
central	$\beta_1 + \beta_2$	+	Relaxation	Bronchodilatation
peripheral	β_2		Relaxation	
Vascular smooth muscle	β_2	+	Relaxation	$\uparrow \dot{V}/\dot{Q}$ mismatch
Endothelium	β_2	+	Inhibition	Anti-permeability
Epithelium	β_2	+		mediators
Mucous glands	β_2	+	Stimulation	
Nerves:	β_2			
prejunctional	β_2	+	Inhibitory	
sensory	β_2	+	Inhibitory	Bronchodilatation
Mast cells	β_2	+	Inhibitory	Reduce mediators
Neutrophils	β_2			
Lymphocytes	β_2			
Cholinergic				
airway smooth muscle,				
central > peripheral	M3	+	Stimulatory	Bronchoconstriction
Submucosal glands	M3 + M1	+	Stimulatory	$\uparrow$ Secretions
Postganglionic nerves	M2	–	Inhibitory	Limit M3 effects
Airway ganglia	M1	+	Stimulatory	Bronchoconstriction

The clinical relevance of other potential effects (Table 5.2) is unclear. Minor effects of β_2 agonists on ciliary function in vitro, and on radiolabelled particulate clearance in vivo have been clearly demonstrated. However, longer-term studies are not available and it is doubtful if clinically significant effects on mucociliary clearance occur. Similarly, although β_2 agonists and anticholinergics might be expected to modulate pathways involved in the cough reflex and small, rather inconsistent, effects on cough challenges have been shown, neither effectively reduces cough symptoms in patients.

'Anti-inflammatory' effects of β_2 agonists (particularly long-acting) are hotly debated. No clinically significant effects on vascular permeability or oedema or airway wall thickness have yet been demonstrated in patients.

Dose–response data

The effect of bronchodilators in COPD is usually assessed as change in FEV_1 or even PEF. There are various reasons why this may be inappropriate scientifically: the disease is defined in terms of limited reversibility, there is wide inter- and intra-individual variation, it is not clear that symptomatic benefit relates particularly well to FEV_1 rather than any other measure of airway function. It can be argued that a dynamic assessment, e.g., walk test or health performance status, quality of life or symptom score, might be better. Construction of dose–responses to β_2 or other drugs is almost impossible in COPD. This bedevils drug comparisons and has an important clinical impact when it comes to evaluation of high-dose inhaled bronchodilators, in particular nebuliser therapy. Small increases in FEV_1 may produce large changes in symptomatic benefit. In fact there is little high-quality comparison data of this kind. A full discussion of nebulised therapy is beyond the scope of this chapter.

Side-effects

At conventional doses the usual minor adverse effects of inhaled β_2 agonists occur in COPD. On the one hand, older patients have fewer β_2 receptors but, on the other, they have been thought to be more sensitive to side-effects. Significant tremor, palpitations, headaches, hypokalaemia or other metabolic effects are uncommon and, although this population of elderly smokers is prone to ischaemic heart disease, exacerbation of angina or significant dysrhythmias are rare.

Anticholinergic agents

This class of inhaled bronchodilators has historically been considered to be more effective than β_2 agonists in patients with COPD and as a consequence, is used by many (especially in North America) as first-line bronchodilator therapy (American Thoracic Society 1995; Barnes 1998). Until now non-selective muscarinic receptor antagonists have been used, but, with advances in pharmacology, new agents have

Table 5.3 Types of muscarinic receptor antagonists

Name	Receptor type
Ipratropium	Non-selective
Oxitropium	Non-selective
Tiotropium	M2 (rapid dissociation), M1 & M3 (slow dissociation)
Darifenacin	M3
Rispenzipine	M1 & M3
Revatropate	M1 & M3

been developed (Table 5.3) which may offer additional therapeutic benefits (Barnes 1998).

Mechanism of action

Binding of acetylcholine to muscarinic (M3) receptors activates rapid hydrolysis of phosphoinositol and formation of inositol-1,4,5-triphosphate (mediated via M3 sites) (Barnes 1987). This leads to release of calcium ions from intracellular stores. Inhibition of adenylyl cyclase reduces cAMP concentrations in airway smooth muscle (mediated via M2 receptors) potentially reducing the effect of β_2-agonist stimulation (Figure 5.1). Muscarinic receptor antagonists act by blocking these receptors within the airways (Barnes 1993, 1998). Five different receptor subtypes have been cloned and functionally identified in humans and animals (Table 5.3). M1 and M3 receptors are excitatory and augment ganglionic nicotinic receptors. M2 receptors are located pre-junctionally at parasympathetic ganglia and nerve terminals; activation inhibits acetylcholine release.

Cholinergic nerves form the dominant bronchoconstrictor pathway in humans. Postganglionic fibres innervate airway smooth muscle, bronchial vessels and submucosal glands, mainly in large airways (Barnes 1987). Activation of these pathways is initiated by sensory afferents in airway epithelium, larynx and nasopharynx (Calverley & Pride 1995) producing reflex bronchoconstriction and maintaining a degree of bronchomotor tone. This has little effect on airway calibre in normal individuals. However, as airway resistance is increased in proportion to the fourth power of airway narrowing, anticholinergic drugs reduce vagal tone and reflex bronchoconstriction more significantly in COPD. This supports the importance of increased vagal tone as a principal component of airway obstruction in COPD (Barnes 1993). As competitive antagonists, the effect of anticholinergic agents depends on the dose until maximum blockade is achieved.

However, reversal of vagal tone on airway smooth muscle may not account entirely for the improvement in lung function. Mucus secretion is under cholinergic control via stimulation of submucosal glands in the large airways (in humans) and from epithelial goblet cells in peripheral airways in human and animal studies in vitro (Rogers *et al.* 1989). The possibility exists that anticholinergics may also improve airflow obstruction by reducing mucus secretion.

Clinical studies

Anticholinergics versus short-acting β_2 agonists

Anticholinergic drugs are at least as effective as, if not more so than, β_2 agonists in improving lung function and symptoms in COPD. As the latter act as physiological antagonists to relax airway smooth muscle this favours an additional non-smooth muscle relaxing effect of anticholinergics, e.g., on mucus secretion (Barnes 1998). Inhaled anticholinergics have a slower onset of action in comparison to short-acting β_2 agonists, but their duration of action (particularly oxitropium) is significantly longer (depending on dose, up to eight hours compared with approximately four hours). Clinical advantages include longer symptom relief and potentially bronchoprotection against a fall in lung function overnight when vagal tone increases (Table 5.4). Significant improvements in spirometry and exercise performance have been demonstrated when compared with placebo (O'Donnell *et al.* 1999).

Rennard *et al.* (1996) performed a retrospective analysis of seven clinical trials, which compared ipratropium with either salbutamol (five studies) or metaproterenol (orciprenaline, two studies) over a 90-day treatment period. The 1,445 patients had moderate to severe COPD (baseline FEV_1 1.0 l). Ipratropium significantly improved baseline lung function; FEV_1 and forced vital capacity (FVC) increased (by 28 and 131 ml respectively) whilst no significant change occurred over time with short-acting β_2 agonists. There was a non-significant decline in the β_2 agonist group after three months. Braun and Levy (1999) produced similar findings.

Intriguing observations of a possible non-bronchodilator effect of ipratropium in delaying an exacerbation of COPD require further study (Friedman 1996; Mahler *et al.* 1999).

Anticholinergics versus long-acting β_2 agonists

Although anticholinergic agents may be more effective than short-acting β_2 agonists, trials comparing ipratropium with long-acting agents such as salmeterol have found the reverse. Mahler *et al.* (1999) reported significantly better lung function in patients randomised to salmeterol ($n = 135$) rather than to ipratropium ($n = 133$) after 12 weeks of treatment (Table 5.4).

Clinical role

Currently inhaled anticholinergic drugs are established as second-line bronchodilators in the management of COPD. Only ipratropium and oxitropium bromide (non-selective anti-muscarinics) are available. There is little to choose between them, although

Table 5.4 Comparison of anticholinergic drugs with inhaled short- and long-acting β_2 agonists

Study	n	Comparison	Baseline $FEV_1(l)$	ΔFEV_1 (ml)	Symptom scores	Comments
Combivent Aerosol Study 1994	534	Ipra (21 μg qds) Salb (100 μg qds) Ipra + Salb	1.0 1.0 1.0	303 305 373*	No significant difference between groups	DBRCT 12-week study
Rennard et al. 1996	1445	Ipra vs β_2 agonist+	1.0 1.0	28* 1	No significant difference between groups	Meta-analysis of 7 clinical trials
Cazzola et al. 1998	16	Oxi (200 μg) Efm (24 μg) Sm (50 μg) Placebo	1.06	230 p 340 p* 270 p 50	– – – –	Single dose study
Mahler et al. 1999	411	Ipra (36 μg qds) Sm (42 μg bd) Placebo	1.16 1.28 1.30	100 p 180 p* 25	Significant decrease in nighttime SOB in sm group	DBRCT 12-week study

KEY

Ipra – ipratropium
Oxi – oxitropium
Salb – salbutamol
Sm – salmeterol
Efm – eformoterol

DBRCT – Double-blind randomised control trial
+ – salbutamol or metaproterenol (orciprenaline)
p – statistically significant vs placebo
* – statistically significant vs other treatment groups
SOB – shortness of breath

oxitropium has a slightly longer duration of action. Although very safe, they are not popular with many patients because of a bitter taste, lack of appreciation of effect (slow onset of action) and the need for regular therapy.

Future role

These drugs produce bronchodilatation by blocking M1 and M3 receptors. Unfortunately they also antagonise presynaptic M2 receptors promoting acetylcholine release, which may tend to overcome M1/M3 blockade. This limits the efficacy of these non-selective agents. To overcome this more selective agents are being developed. Tiotropium bromide is an example. This drug exhibits kinetic selectivity, rapidly dissociating from M2 receptors and slowly dissociating from M1 and M3 receptors (Barnes 2000). This produces prolonged bronchodilatation for up to 24 hours in COPD patients (Littner *et al.* 2000). It is inhaled once daily with benefits in terms of prophylaxis and compliance. It is well tolerated and offers the opportunity to realise the full pharmacological potential of this class of agents in routine clinical practice (Calverley 2000). Potentially it could also be combined with an inhaled long-acting β_2 agonist.

Other, new, highly selective M1/M3 antagonists such as revatropate and darifenacin are in development and may eventually be used in treating COPD.

Long-acting inhaled β_2 agonists

Conventional short-acting β_2 agonists have been used for many years as first-line treatment of patients with chronic airflow obstruction. Over the last decade, the development of long-acting β_2 agents has raised questions over their place in the treatment of COPD.

Salmeterol and eformoterol are now firmly established in the treatment of asthma as they improve symptoms, lung function and are also broncho-protective. However, neither the American Thoracic Society (ATS) nor the British Thoracic Society (BTS) guidelines have clarified their use in COPD (Ulrik 1995). The main advantage of these agents is their long duration of action (about 12 hours), potentially giving them an important role in maintenance therapy before other agents such as oral methylxanthines (Cazzola & Matera 1999). A number of studies (Appleton *et al.* 1999) now support their use in this way (Table 5.5).

Salmeterol

Salmeterol was the first inhaled long-acting agent to be introduced. It is a lipophilic compound with a duration of action of approximately 12 hours. Onset of action is approximately 20 minutes and it has a peak effect at approximately 4–6 hours. Common side-effects include tremor, headache, sweating, palpitations and tachycardia/arrhythmias. Tolerance has not been demonstrated in COPD.

Table 5.5 Comparison of long-acting β_2 agonists with other bronchodilators

Study	n	Comparison	Baseline $FEV_1(l)$	ΔFEV_1 (ml)	Comments
Ulrik et al. 1995	63	Sm 50 µg bd Placebo	1.21 1.24	50 10	DBRCT decrease in day/ night symptoms in Sm group
Boyd et al. 1997	674	Sm 50 µg bd Sm 100 µg bd Placebo	1.31 1.23 1.31	70 * 90 * −20	DBRCT
Jones et al. 1997	283	Sm 50 µg bd Sm 100 µg bd Placebo	1.40 1.40 1.30	117 * 100 * 27	DBRCT Improved SGRQ in Sm groups
van Noord et al. 2000	144	Sm 50 µg bd Sm 50 µg bd+ Ipra 40 µg qds placebo	1.30 1.40 1.30	65 * 112 *† 13	DBRCT reduction in symptoms in Sm groups
Cazzola & Santangelo et al. 1994	16	Sm 50 µg Efm 24 µg Salb 200 µg Placebo	1.04 1.13 1.02 1.10	332 402 399	Single-dose 12-h study
Cazzola & Matera et al. 1995	12	Sm 25, 50, 75 µg Efm 12, 24, 36 µg	Range: 0.25–0.98	Significant increases in FEV_1 in all groups‡	Single-dose 12-h study

KEY:
Sm – salmeterol
Efm – eformoterol
Salb – salbutamol
Ipra – ipratropium

DRBCT = double-blind randomised controlled trial
6MW = 6-minute walk test
* Statistically significant vs placebo
† Statistically significant vs other treatment groups
‡ Greatest response in patients taking eformoterol 36 µg and salmeterol 50 µg

The efficacy:side-effect dose–response favours a maximum dose of salmeterol 50 μg bd to minimise side-effects.

Clinical studies

Initial studies compared salmeterol with placebo in moderate to severe COPD. One such double-blind, randomised, crossover trial compared salmeterol 50 μg with placebo, each twice daily, over four weeks (Ulrik 1995). This showed a significant improvement in symptom scores and morning PEF in the salmeterol arm of the study. However, no difference was found in spirometry and the trial was of short duration. Boyd et al. (1997) carried out a similar, larger, parallel group study comparing salmeterol 50 and 100 μg bd with placebo over 16 weeks. Symptoms (and reduced use of short-acting β_2 agonists) were better in those using salmeterol and FEV_1 was improved by approximately 7 per cent. Exercise tolerance, as assessed by the six-minute walk test, was unchanged. The 100 μg dose was associated with increased side-effects.

Other studies have focused specifically on symptom scores and used methods such as the St George's Respiratory Questionnaire (SGRQ) in comparison with spirometric assessment. Jones and Bosh (1997) compared salmeterol 50 and 100 μg bd with placebo in the Boyd study. Patients were well matched in terms of baseline FEV_1. Significant improvement in SGRQ was seen in the 50 μg bd group but not at 100 μg due to side-effects. This was mirrored by a modest increase in FEV_1 (approximately 180 ml), showing that slight changes in lung function can produce significant symptomatic benefit.

These clinical and physiological benefits have been observed when compared with other bronchodilators such as anticholinergics. Studies comparing salmeterol and ipratropium have already been mentioned. Single administration of salmeterol produced greater sustained bronchodilatation over 12 hours (as measured by FEV_1 area under the curve [AUC]) than ipratropium given four times a day (Mahler et al. 1999). Benefit from salmeterol has been demonstrated in COPD patients of all severities (Donohue et al. 1999).

Salmeterol has also been shown to improve ciliary function and to decrease epithelial cell damage on exposure to toxins produced by *Pseudomonas aeruginosa* in vitro (Dowling et al. 1997, 1999). These effects on *Pseudomonas aeruginosa*, a known opportunistic coloniser of airways in severe COPD, may relate to increasing time to onset of a COPD exacerbation (Fagon & Chastre 1996).

Eformoterol

Eformoterol is a newer long-acting agent with well-established therapeutic benefit in the treatment of asthma. Reduced lipophilicity compared with salmeterol results in slightly different pharmacological properties: a faster onset of action (approximately 2–3 minutes compared with 20 minutes for salmeterol); a slightly earlier peak effect at approximately four hours (cf. six hours) but with a similar duration of action at 12 hours. Its side-effect profile is similar to that of other β_2 agonists.

Clinical studies

Eformoterol is not currently recommended for the treatment of COPD but studies show potential benefit. Two studies compared eformoterol (12–24 µg), salmeterol (25, 50 and 75 µg), salbutamol (200 µg) and placebo in groups consisting of 12 and 16 moderate–severe COPD patients respectively (Cazzola *et al.* 1994, 1995). Both were single-dose studies showing significant improvement in FEV_1 and overall bronchodilatation (duration and clinical effect) with the long-acting agents when compared with salbutamol or placebo. There was also a dose–response with eformoterol, which was absent with salmeterol.

Another study compared eformoterol and ipratropium in terms of efficacy and safety (Dahl *et al.* 2000). Seven hundred and eighty patients were randomised to receive eformoterol (either 12 or 24 µg bd), ipratropium (40 µg qds) or placebo for a period of 12 weeks. All treatment groups produced significant improvements in FEV_1 AUC compared with placebo but eformoterol at either dose was significantly better than ipratropium. A similar number of adverse events were seen in all four groups. Clearly long-term comparisons are needed to evaluate effectiveness.

Clinical role

Salmeterol and eformoterol have an evolving clinical role in the management of COPD. Larger, long-term, comparative studies are necessary for true evaluation of their place in guidelines. Both are available in a variety of devices but both are considerably more expensive than conventional short-acting agents. There is no evidence favouring their use concomitant with nebulised β_2 agonist therapy.

Theophyllines

This class of drugs has been used in patients with COPD and asthma for over 50 years. However, in the UK the theophyllines have moved from being first-line to becoming third- or even fourth-line therapy (Ramsdell 1995). This is due to the development of new, more effective, inhaled bronchodilators, together with their side-effect profile. Furthermore, despite a variety of slow-release preparations, it may be difficult to achieve adequate, therapeutic plasma concentrations in individual patients. Benefit is modest, however, and their clinical effects may not be solely accounted for by bronchodilatation. High-quality evidence is surprisingly sparse probably because the drugs are old and cheap. Table 5.6 includes a number of small studies of theophylline demonstrating an additive effect when used together with inhaled bronchodilators, particularly in terms of spirometry and exercise capacity (Clark & Boyd 1980; Taylor *et al.* 1985; Dullinger *et al.* 1986; Tandon & Kailis 1991; Nishimura *et al.* 1993).

Table 5.6 Summary of clinical evidence for combination therapy with oral theophyllines

Study	n	Comparison	Mean baseline FEV_1 (l)	Mean baseline FCV (l)	ΔFEV_1 (ml)	ΔFVC (ml)	Comments
Taylor et al. 1985	25	Theo (bd) [a]	1.15	2.50	120*	190*	DBRXOCT 4 treatment periods, each 3 weeks' duration
		Salb (200 µg qds)			70*	240*	
		Theo + Salb			230**	520**	
		Placebo			−10	50	
Nishimura et al. 1993	12	Theo [b]	0.92	2.94	290*	170*	DBRXOCT. No significant differences between groups
		Placebo			250	70	
Guyatt et al. 1989	19	Theo/placebo	1.02	2.73		−140	DBRXOCT 4 treatment periods, each 2 weeks' duration
		Salb/placebo				20 *	
		Theo/Salb				150 *	
		Placebo				−370	
Murciano et al. 1989	60	Theo (10 mg/kg)	31.5%[c]	60.1%[c]	+13%[d]	+10%[d]	DBRXOCT Significant decrease in dyspnoea score in Theo group
		Placebo	31.6%[c]	59.5%[c]	−2%[d]	−4%[d]	

KEY

Theo – theophylline
Salb – salbutamol

[a] Sustained release preparation, dose determined by plasma levels
[b] 400 mg for 2 weeks then 600 mg for a further 2 weeks
[c] Values expressed as percentage predicted FEV_1 and FVC
[d] Values expressed as percentage of baseline FEV_1 and FVC
* Statistically significant vs placebo
** Statistically significant vs placebo and vs other treatment groups
DBRXOCT – double-blind, randomised, crossover control trial

Mechanism of action

The classic mechanism of action is that of phosphodiesterase (PDE) inhibition increasing cAMP concentrations by inhibiting breakdown. However, other mechanisms may be involved.

Phosphodiesterase inhibition

Both aminophylline and theophylline are non-selective PDE inhibitors with in vitro inhibitory effects on neutrophil function, in particular chemotaxis, activation, degranulation and adherence (Aubier & Barnes 1995). Theophyllines increase levels of intracellular cAMP but there is no evidence to suggest preferential concentration of these drugs in smooth muscle cells, and relaxation of human airway smooth muscle is poor at measured plasma therapeutic concentrations.

An increasing number of PDE isoenzymes have been identified in various human tissues (Soderling & Beavo 2000). The PDE-4 and PDE-3 subtypes are currently thought to be the most important in lung as they are present in bronchial smooth muscle and also inflammatory cells. PDE-4 modulation influences neutrophil function and mediates release of chemotactic factors from alveolar macrophages (Beavo 1995). It is not clear to what extent specific PDE-4 inhibitors may influence the inflammatory process in COPD.

Adenosine receptor inhibition

At therapeutic concentrations, theophylline acts as a potent inhibitor of adenosine receptors, which could theoretically produce bronchodilatation. Bronchoconstriction induced by inhaled adenosine was prevented by inhaled theophylline in asthmatics (Cushley *et al.* 1984).

Immunomodulation

In vivo there is limited evidence for an immunomodulatory action of theophyllines, inhibition of mast cells, stimulation of suppressor CD8+ T cells (Dullinger *et al.* 1986), etc.

Pharmacokinetics

Theophylline is rapidly and totally absorbed from the gastrointestinal tract. Clearance varies considerably between patients, so individual dosing regimens are required with close dose monitoring of plasma concentration. A therapeutic range of 10–20 mg/l is recommended to achieve a clinical response with the least risk of side-effects, but evidence for this in COPD is scant (Milgrom & Bender 1993). Metabolism occurs in the liver predominantly by the cytochrome P450/P448 microsomal enzyme system, which is influenced by a variety of factors (Troger & Meyer 1995). Metabolism is increased by cigarette smoking, co-administration of enzyme inducers, e.g., anticonvulsants such as phenytoin and carbamazepine. Other drugs reduce metabolism: these include antibiotics (e.g., erythromycin, some quinolones) and cimetidine by inhibiting cytochrome P450. Other factors that reduce hepatic metabolism include ageing, liver disease, heart failure, pneumonia and certain vaccinations (Milgrom & Bender 1993).

Adverse effects

Theophylline has a narrow toxic:therapeutic ratio, especially in elderly patients (Taylor *et al.* 1985). Considerable potential for side-effects exists especially with long-term use. Most adverse effects arise through increased dosing but inadequate monitoring of plasma levels and reduced metabolism through co-administration of other drugs may contribute. Recognised side-effects include arrhythmias, headaches, insomnia and gastrointestinal symptoms, hypo- or hyperkalaemia, and convulsions (Milgrom & Bender 1993). Theophylline is poorly tolerated in some individuals even at low doses (and low plasma levels).

Clinical benefit

Chronic therapy is associated with an improvement in lung function, FEV_1, VC and minute ventilation, and a reduction in hyperinflation (Murciano *et al.* 1989). Potentially theophylline may also increase diaphragm muscle strength, delay the onset of fatigue and stimulate ciliary function as well as stimulating respiratory drive, improving cardiac function and reducing pulmonary artery pressure. All of these effects may contribute to an improvement of functional capacity.

Future role

Specific PDE inhibitors are under development and one study suggests surprisingly impressive benefit with SB 207499 (Ariflo), a second-generation PDE-4 inhibitor (Torphy *et al.* 1999).

Oral β_2 agonists

Oral preparations of β_2 agonists, including salbutamol, terbutaline and bambuterol, are used infrequently in the UK. The ATS and BTS guidelines (ATS 1995; BTS 1997) give different advice. The American guidelines suggest that oral agents such as salbutamol may be used if combined inhaled therapies fail to control symptoms (particularly at night). However, it is clearly stated that there is no formal evidence supporting this use. The BTS guidelines do not advocate their use at all. Only very rarely is it justified to prescribe an oral β_2 agonist because it is not possible to find an inhaler device that a particular patient can use. The main problems are those of variable plasma concentrations and significant side-effects, e.g., arrhythmias, myocardial insufficiency and hypokalaemia.

Leukotriene receptor antagonists

Two Cys-LT1 receptor antagonists are curently available in the UK: montelukast and zafirlukast. Although leukotriene-modifying drugs might be anticipated to be effective in a condition involving neutrophilic inflammation, no controlled evidence of efficacy in COPD has been published.

Combination therapy

As a general pharmacological principle it is often advantageous to combine low doses of two or more drugs with different mechanisms of action. Beneficial effects may be additive or even greater with reduced adverse/side-effects compared to high doses of a single agent.

Combination of inhaled bronchodilators

Since β_2 agonists and anticholinergic agents produce bronchodilatation by different mechanisms (acting on receptors distributed differently in the bronchial tree, Figure 5.1) it is logical to combine inhaled therapy. Besides producing a greater bronchodilator effect than either agent alone, the rapid onset of action of a β_2 agonist with the greater duration of an anticholinergic agent is an additional rationale. Furthermore, given by a single combination inhaler, there are additional benefits of simplicity, reduced cost and potentially enhanced compliance. The European Respiratory Society (ERS), BTS and ATS guidelines also suggest a role for long-acting β_2 agonists in combination with anticholinergic drugs in chronic stable disease (ATS 1995; Siafakas *et al.* 1995; BTS 1997).

The best evidence for β_2-agonist/anticholinergic combination therapy has emerged over the last decade. The Combivent Inhalation Aerosol Study Group (1994) randomised 534 patients with moderate to severe COPD (mean baseline FEV_1 1.3 l) to either salbutamol 50 µg bd, salbutamol 50 µg bd plus ipratropium 40 mg qds (in a single inhaler device) or placebo. At 12 weeks there was at least a 30 per cent improvement in mean FEV_1 and FVC with the combination therapy compared to 24–27 per cent for those using monotherapy. Importantly there was no change in side-effects. Another study showed a reduction in exacerbation events in those patients using Combivent when compared with monotherapy (Friedman *et al.* 1996).

Similar clinical benefit has also been demonstrated combining ipratropium bromide and other short-acting β_2 agonists. Duovent is a much older combination inhaler containing ipratropium with fenoterol. This produced greater improvement in lung function compared with monotherapy (Morton 1984; Serra & Giacopelli 1986; LeDoux *et al.* 1989). However, Imhof *et al.* (1996) compared Duovent, salbutamol and placebo in 24 patients with COPD and found that Duovent and salbutamol produced similar maximal increases in FEV_1 and decreases in specific airway resistance, although these differences were significantly greater than placebo.

In clinical practice, combination therapy is established and two main formulations are used: Combivent (ipratropium bromide + salbutamol) and Duovent (ipratropium bromide + fenoterol). Both therapies may be given by metered dose inhaler (one to two puffs, three to four times daily) or as a nebuliser solution. Peak effect occurs at approximately 30–60 minutes post-dose and may last 4–6 hours. Both are well tolerated but concerns persist regarding the use of Duovent due to its fenoterol component (Imhof *et al.* 1993; Beasley *et al.* 1999). Combivent is preferred but both are relatively expensive.

Long-acting β_2 agonists and anticholinergics in combination

Following the proven benefits of adding short-acting β_2 agonists to anticholinergics, various studies have examined the combination of long-acting β_2 agonists and anticholinergics (Mahler *et al.* 1999; van Noord *et al.* 2000).

Most studies have used salmeterol in conjunction with ipratropium bromide in stable COPD. Van Noord *et al.* (2000) studied 144 patients (mean baseline FEV_1 0.99 l) randomised to treatment with salmeterol alone, salmeterol and ipratropium or placebo for a period of 12 weeks. The greatest increase in FEV_1 occurred in those using combination therapy (8 per cent rise) compared with the salbutamol (5 per cent) and placebo (1 per cent) groups. Clearly, long-term studies involving larger patient numbers and subjects with a broader spectrum of disease severity are needed to evaluate the true benefits. Eformoterol has shown similar clinical benefits to salmeterol in COPD patients and requires assessment in combination with anticholinergic therapy (Cazzola *et al.* 1994). The most recent BTS guidelines suggest that long-acting β_2 agonists are best used in those individuals with a bronchodilator response to short-acting β_2 agonists and where inhaled short-acting β_2 agonists and anticholinergics have failed to control symptoms. There is minimal evidence to support this. Long-acting β_2 agonists should be tried in everyone but only continued if there is a genuine improvement in symptoms or lung function. With the development of more selective and longer-acting anticholinergics, combination therapy with long-acting β_2 agonists may offer better symptom control with reduced dosing and improved compliance.

Theophyllines in combination therapy

Although initially used as monotherapy 50 years ago, theophyllines are now considered a third- or fourth-line treatment in patients already taking inhaled bronchodilators (usually a β_2 agonist plus an anticholinergic) (Ramsdell 1995). Scientific evidence regarding this role is surprisingly sparse. Cynics might argue that theophylline is cheap and no pharmaceutical company has a monopoly. Most studies have concentrated on combining theophylline with a β_2 agonist and results have shown either an additive effect (Taylor *et al.* 1985; Guyatt *et al.* 1987) or no significant benefit (Clark & Boyd 1980; Dullinger *et al.* 1986; Tandon & Kailis

1991; Nishimura *et al.* 1993) (Table 5.6). Overall it appears that theophylline offers some additional benefit in particular individuals, but it is unclear if this applies to very high doses of inhaled therapy.

Bronchodilators in outpatient management of COPD patients

Acute: assessment of bronchodilator response reversibility testing

Although this is generally recommended (ATS 1995; Siafakas *et al.* 1995; BTS 1997) the reasons are not particularly clear. It can sometimes be useful to distinguish asthma from COPD. More often it may rapidly demonstrate an asthmatic component in mixed disease. Practice varies from unit to unit. Administration of salbutamol, together with ipratropium, separately or sequentially, usually by nebuliser to circumvent difficulties with inhaler devices and 'submaximal dosing' (using 2.5 mg and 0.5 mg respectively) can be used to document immediate reversibility. This may have value for characterising a patient, e.g., for inclusion in a clinical trial. However, it is well known that this is poorly reproducibile day to day (Anthonisen *et al.* 1983; Calverley & Pride 1995). It may define maximum achievable values but may be better performed following a 'steroid trial'. For the reasons outlined above, acute comparison of different drug doses by different inhaler devices or a nebuliser may be misleading (see Dose–response data, p 46).

Chronic: sequential trials of therapy

In clinical practice management of individual patients involves sequential 'trials of one'. Treatments, usually in combination, are given aimed at minimising symptoms and optimising FEV_1 and quality of life. It is important that treatments producing no objective or subjective benefit are stopped. However, reassessment at a later stage may be justified. Assessing outcome and cost–benefit at an individual patient level is a major challenge.

Delivery of care

The involvement of respiratory care nurses (RCNs) in the management of COPD, building on previous work in asthma, should be encouraged. Choosing the appropriate inhaler device, optimising its use, adjusting inhaled bronchodilator doses, conducting sequential trials of therapy according to protocols, monitoring progress and organising nebuliser therapy (Nebuliser Project Group, BTS 1997) all fall within the remit of an RCN in general practice.

Current guidelines

At present three sets of guidelines from the BTS, ATS and ERS are available on the management of COPD. There is a general consensus on treatment except for a few variations (Table 5.7).

Table 5.7 Current and proposed guidelines for bronchodilator therapy in COPD

Treatment step	Current management guidelines			Proposed guidelines
	ATS	BTS	ERS	
1st	Inhaled short-acting β_2 agonists or anticholinergic	Inhaled short-acting β_2 agonists		Inhaled short-acting β_2 agonists
2nd	Inhaled anticholinergic*	Inhaled anticholinergic		Inhaled anticholinergic and β_2 combination
3rd	Oral theophylline or oral β_2 agonists	Oral theophylline preparation		Inhaled long-acting β_2 agonists
4th	Inhaled long-acting β_2 agonists[†]			Oral theophylline
5th	[#] Nebuliser therapy			

KEY
* If not already used by the patient
[†] Only if nocturnal symptoms present or positive bronchodilator response to inhaled β_2 agonists
[#] Only if tolerant to other therapies

Proposed guidelines

In the light of current clinical evidence we make further recommendations. The principal differences are the regular use of long-acting β_2 agonists with anticholinergics if symptom control is inadequate. The potential benefits may be greater once long-acting selective anticholinergics are available. Each step only follows if there is documented benefit but subjective effects are weighted equally with lung function improvements. If addition of an anticholinergic alone is helpful then Combivent is recommended. If nebuliser therapy is used long-acting β_2 agonists are withdrawn.

Summary

Conventional, inhaled, short-acting β_2 agonists are most widely used initially. Anticholinergics, although less popular, should be tried and if objective or subjective benefit is shown they should be continued probably as a combination inhaler. The efficacy of inhaled long-acting β_2 agonists is now established in COPD, although there are no published comparisons of salmeterol and eformoterol. Oral β_2 agonists are little used. Slow-release theophylline preparations retain a place in treating COPD despite intolerance, potential drug interactions and inherent toxicity which requires monitoring of blood levels. A trial of nebuliser therapy is reserved for late-stage disease. Sequential trials of additional therapy are given aimed at minimising symptoms and optimising FEV_1 and quality of life. Attention must be paid to the use of inhalers and delivery of care generally.

References

American Thoracic Society (1995). Standards for the diagnosis and care of patients with chronic obstructive pulmonary disease. *American Journal of Respiratory & Critical Care Medicine* **52**, S77–121

Anthonisen NR, Wright EC, Hodgkin JE *et al.* (1983). Prognosis in chronic obstructive pulmonary disease. *American Review of Respiratory Disease* **136**, 14–20

Appleton S, Smith B, Veale B, Bara A (1999). Regular long acting Beta-2 adrenoceptor agonists in stable chronic obstructive airways disease. *Cochrane Library* **1**

Aubier M & Barnes PJ (1995). Theophylline and phosphodiesterase inhibtors. *European Respiratory Journal* **8**, 347–348

Barnes PJ (1987). Cholinergic control of airway smooth muscle. *American Review of Respiratory Disease* **136**, S42–45

Barnes PJ (1993). Muscarinic receptor subtypes in airways. *Life Sciences* **52**, 521–528

Barnes PJ (1998). New therapies for chronic obstructive pulmonary disease. *Thorax* **53**, 137–47

Barnes PJ (2000).The pharmacological properties of tiotropium. *Chest* **117**, 63S–66S

Beasley R, Pearce N, Crane J, Burgess C (1999). Beta agonists: what is the evidence that their use increases the risk of asthma morbidity and mortality? *Journal of Allergy & Clinical Immunology* **104**, S18–S30

Beavo JA (1995). Cyclic nucleotide phosphodiesterases: functional implications of multiple isoforms. *Physiological Reviews* **75**, 725–748

Boyd G, Morice AH, Pounsford JC, Siebert M, Peslis N, Crawford C (1997). An evaluation of salmeterol in the treatment of chronic obstructive pulmonary disease (COPD). *European Respiratory Journal* **10**, 815–21

Braun SR & Levy SF (1999). Comparison of ipratropium bromide and albuterol in chronic obstructive pulmonary disease: a three-center study. *American Journal of Medicine* **91**, 28S–32S

British Thoracic Society (1997). Guidelines for the management of chronic obstructive pulmonary disease (1997). The COPD Guidelines Group of the Standards of Care Committee of the BTS. *Thorax* **52**, S1–S28

Calverley PMA (2000). The future for tiotropium. *Chest* **117**, 67S–69S

Calverley PMA & Pride NB (1995). *Management of Chronic Obstructive Pulmonary Disease*, 1st edn. London: Chapman & Hall, pp391–445

Cazzola M & Matera MG (1999). Should long-acting beta 2-agonists be considered an alternative first choice option for the treatment of stable COPD? *Respiratory Medicine* **93**, 227–229

Cazzola M, Santangelo G, Piccolo A *et al.* (1994). Effect of salmeterol and formoterol in patients with chronic obstructive pulmonary disease. *Pulmonary Pharmacology* **7**, 103–107

Cazzola M, Matera MG, Santangelo G, Vinciguerra A, Rossi F, D'Amato G (1995). Salmeterol and formoterol in partially reversible severe COPD: a dose-response study. *Respiratory Medicine* **89**, 357–362

Clark CJ & Boyd G (1980). Combination of aminophylline (PhyllocontinContinuus tablets) and salbutamol in the management of chronic obstructive airways disease. *British Journal of Clinical Pharmacology* **9**, 359–64

Combivent Inhalation Aerosol Study Group (1994). In chronic obstructive pulmonary disease, a combination of ipratropium and albuterol is more effective than either agent alone. An 85-day multicenter trial. *Chest* **105**, 411–419

Current Best Practice for Nebuliser Treatment (1997). The Nebuliser Project Group of the British Thoracic Society Standards of Care Committee. *Thorax* **52**, S49–S52

Cushley MJ, Tattersfield AE, Holgate ST (1984). Adenosine-induced bronchoconstriction in asthma. Antagonism by inhaled theophylline. *American Review of Respiratory Disease* **129**, 380–384

Dahl R, Greefhorst APM, Nowak D *et al.* (2000). Comparison of the efficacy and safety in inhaled formoterol and ipratropium in patients with COPD. *American Journal of Respiratory & Critical Care Medicine* **161**, A489

Donohue J, Emmett A, Rickard K, Knobil K (1999). Salmeterol is effective bronchodilator therapy for all stages of COPD. *American Journal of Respiratory & Critical Care Medicine* **159**, A817

Dowling RB, Johnson M, Cole PJ, Wilson R (1999). Effect of fluticasone propionate and salmeterol on Pseudomonas aeruginosa infection of the respiratory mucosa in vitro. *European Respiratory Journal* **14**, 363–369

Dowling RB, Rayner CF, Rutman A *et al.* (1997). Effect of salmeterol on Pseudomonas aeruginosa infection of respiratory mucosa. *American Journal of Respiratory & Critical Care Medicine* **155**, 327–336

Dullinger D, Kronenberg R, Niewoehner DE (1986). Efficacy of inhaled metaproterenol and orally-administered theophylline in patients with chronic airflow obstruction. *Chest* **89**, 171–3

Fagon JY & Chastre J (1996). Severe exacerbations of COPD patients: the role of pulmonary infections. *Seminars in Respiratory Infections* **11**, 109–18

Friedman M (1996). A multicenter study of nebulised bronchodilator solutions in chronic obstructive pulmonary disease. *American Journal of Medicine* **100**, 30S–39S

Friedman M, Witek Jr TJ, Serny CW, Flanders J, Menioge SS, Wilson JD (1996). Combination bronchodilator therapy is associated with a reduction in exacerbations (E) of COPD. *American Journal of Respiratory & Critical Care Medicine* **153**, A126

Guyatt GH, Townsend M, Pugsley SO *et al.* (1987). Bronchodilators in chronic air-flow limitation. Effects on airway function, exercise capacity, and quality of life. *American Review of Respiratory Disease* **135**, 1069–1074

Jones PW & Bosh TK (1997). Quality of life changes in COPD patients treated with salmeterol. *American Journal of Respiratory & Critical Care Medicine* **155**, 1283–1289

Imhof E, Ehasser S, Karrer W *et al.* (1993). Comparison of bronchodilator effects of fenoterol/ipratropium bromide and salbutamol in patients with chronic obstructive lung disease. *Respiration* **60**, 84–88

LeDoux EJ, Morris JF, Temple WP, Duncan C (1989). Standard and double dose ipratropium bromide and combined ipratropium bromide and inhaled metaproterenol in COPD. *Chest* **95**, 1013–1016

Littner MR, Ilowite JS, Tashkin DP *et al.* (2000). Long-acting bronchodilation with once-daily dosing of tiotropium (Spiriva). in stable chronic obstructive pulmonary disease. *American Journal of Respiratory & Critical Care Medicine* **161**, 1136–1142

Mahler DA, Donohue JF, Barbee RA *et al.* (1999). Efficacy of salmeterol xinafoate in the treatment of COPD. *Chest* **115**, 957–965

Milgrom H & Bender B (1993). Current issues in the use of theophylline. *American Review of Respiratory Disease* **147**, S33–S39

Morton O (1984). Response to Duovent of chronic reversible airways obstruction – a controlled trial in general practice. *Postgraduate Medical Journal* **60**, 249–253

Murciano D, Auclair MH, Pariente R, Aubier M (1989). A randomised controlled trial of theophylline in patients with severe chronic obstructive pulmonary disease. *New England Journal of Medicine* **320**, 1521–1525

Nishimura K, Koyama H, Ikeda A, Izumi T (1993). Is oral theophylline effective in combination with both inhaled anticholinergic agent and inhaled beta 2-agonist in the treatment of stable COPD? *Chest* **104**, 179–184

O'Donnell DE, Lam M, Webb KA (1999). Spirometric correlates of improvement in exercise performance after anticholinergic therapy in chronic obstructive pulmonary disease. *American Journal of Respiratory & Critical Care Medicine* **160**, 542–549

Ramsdell J (1995). Use of theophylline in the treatment of COPD. *Chest* **107**, 206S–209S

Rennard SI, Serby CW, Ghafouri M, Johnson PA, Friedman M (1996). Extended therapy with ipratropium is associated with improved lung function in patients with COPD. A retrospective analysis of data from seven clinical trials. *Chest* **110**, 63–67

Rogers DF, Aursudkij B, Barnes PJ (1989). Effects of tachykinins on mucus secretion on human bronchi in vitro. *European Journal of Pharmacology* **174**, 283–286

Serra C & Giacopelli A (1986). Controlled clinical study of a long-term treatment of chronic obstructive lung disease using a combination of fenoterol and ipratropium bromide in aerosol form. *Respiration* **50**, 249–253

Siafakas NM, Vermeire P, Pride NB *et al.* (1995). Optimal assessment and management of chronic obstructive pulmonary disease (COPD). The European Respiratory Society Task Force. *European Respiratory Journal* **8**, 1398–1420

Soderling SH & Beavo JA (2000). Regulation of cAMP and cGMP signaling: new phosphodiesterase and new functions. *Current Opinion in Cell Biology* **12**, 174–179

Tandon MK & Kailis SG (1991). Bronchodilator treatment for partially reversible chronic obstructive airways disease. *Thorax* **46**, 248–251

Taylor DR, Buick B, Kinney C, Lowry RC, McDevitt DG (1985). The efficacy of orally administered theophylline, inhaled salbutamol, and a combination of the two as chronic therapy in the management of chronic bronchitis with reversible air-flow obstruction. *American Review of Respiratory Disease* **131**, 747–751

Torphy TJ, Barnette MS, Underwood DC *et al.* (1999). Ariflo (SB 207499), a second generation phosphodiesterase 4 inhibitor for the treatment and COPD: from concept to clinic. *Pulmonary Pharmacology & Therapeutics* **12**, 131–135

Troger U & Meyer FP (1995). Influence of endogenous and exogenous effectors on the pharmacokinetics of theophylline. Focus on biotransformation. *Clinical Pharmacokinetics* **28**, 287–314

Ulrik CS (1995). Efficacy of inhaled salmeterol in the management of smokers with COPD: a single centre randomised, double blind, placebo controlled, crossover study. *Thorax* **50**, 750–754

van Noord JA, de Munck DR, Bantje TA, Hop WC, Akveld ML, Bommer AM (2000). Long-term treatment of chronic obstructive pulmonary disease with salmeterol and the additive effect of ipratropium. *European Respiratory Journal* **15**, 878–885

Chapter 6

Scientific evidence and expert clinical opinion for the selection and use of inhaled corticosteroids in the treatment of chronic obstructive pulmonary disease

P Sherwood Burge

Introduction

The history of corticosteroid use in patients with chronic obstructive pulmonary disease (COPD) has been based on an inadequate understanding of the disease, which includes lung destruction (emphysema) and irreversible sclerosis of small airways (obliterative bronchitis), as well as some larger airway inflammation. It is generally progressive. Early studies tried to separate responders from non-responders and base treatment on this separation. There are no studies showing a different outcome with long-term corticosteroid treatment based on this separation. One study using a blinded placebo-controlled steroid trial, but an open follow-up, showed absolutely no difference in forced expiratory volume in 1 second (FEV_1) decline between responders and non-responders (Weir *et al.* 1994), but a significant effect of inhaled beclomethasone on subsequent FEV_1 decline. Newer studies have recognised that the disease is progressive, and that slowing its rate of progression is the most realistic outcome for non-surgical treatment. Inhaled corticosteroids have been used widely for patients with COPD in advance of any studies showing long-term efficacy. Small early studies often included subjects with definite asthma as well as COPD (the separation is often difficult in patients with severe disease because of the non-pathological definitions of the diseases). Three smaller studies have been re-analysed using a common entry definition with exclusion of asthmatics (van Grunsven *et al.* 1999). A further medium size study (Weir *et al.* 1999), a large six-month study (Paggiaro *et al.* 1998) and four large studies (the Copenhagen City Lung Study [Vestbo *et al.* 1999], Euroscop [Pauwels *et al.* 1999], Isolde [Burge *et al.* 2000] and Lung Health-2 [Lung Health Study Research Group 2000]) lasting at least three years have been published. All these studies were randomised, double blind and placebo controlled. A population based study has also linked treatment after hospital discharge following an exacerbation of COPD with re-admissions and deaths over the following year (Sin & Tu 2001). There is now sufficient evidence to recommend the use of inhaled corticosteroids in patients with COPD.

Who has been studied?

The entry demographics for the main studies are shown in Table 6.1. Patients for the Copenhagen City Lung Study were recruited from a random population sample and included all those 30–70 years old with a reduced FEV_1/FVC ratio (FVC = forced vital capacity), irrespective of their actual FEV_1 value, who failed to respond to an oral steroid and bronchodilator trial (Vestbo et al. 1999). They constitute the most mildly affected group and few of them are likely to develop sufficiently severe disease to die prematurely of respiratory failure.

Table 6.1 Demographics of intention-to-treat populations in the main studies referenced (means)

	Isolde	Meta-analysis	Exacerbation	Weir	Lung Health-2	Euroscop	Copenhagen
FEV_1 (litres)	1.4	1.36	1.56	1.1	2.1	2.5	2.4
FEV_1 (% predicted)	50	45	57	40	64	77	86
FEV_1/FVC	44	48	57	38	57	62	56
Age	64	61	63	67	56	52	59
Smokers (%)	48	63	49	36	90	100	76

Their FEV_1 was above 100 per cent predicted in 22 per cent and above 80 per cent predicted in 61 per cent. Their mean age was 59. Euroscop studied an intermediate group who had to be smokers who failed a smoking cessation programme during the first three months of the study, and were generally recruited by advertisement rather than from clinic populations (Pauwels et al. 1999). They constitute the group in whom intervention is most likely to lead to long-term benefit. The study, however, had FEV_1 decline as its only usable outcome measure. Lung Health-2 recruited subjects who had completed Lung Health-1 and continued to smoke. Lung Health-1 attempted to recruit healthy smokers. However, the group contained many with definite COPD, a group intermediate in severity between Euroscop and Isolde. Isolde mainly recruited patients from hospital clinics, and are the most severely affected of the main studies (Burge et al. 2000). The smaller studies are of similar patients (van Grunsven et al. 1999; Weir et al. 1999), as was the six-month study designed specifically to investigate the role of inhaled steroids on disease exacerbations (the patients were recruited as frequent exacerbators) (Paggiaro et al. 1998). A large study of more than 20,000 hospital discharges, following an exacerbation of COPD in Ontario, Canada, linked specific drug prescribing, including the use of inhaled corticosteroids, with centrally collected admission and mortality data (Sin & Tu 2000).

Doses of inhaled steroid used

The studies showing the greatest benefit have used the highest doses of inhaled corticosteroids. The Isolde (Burge *et al.* 2000), Weir *et al.* (1999) and Exacerbation (Paggiaro *et al.* 1998) studies used fluticasone propionate 1 mg/day or beclomethasone dipropionate 2 mg/day. Euroscop (Pauwels *et al.* 1999) and the Copenhagen City Lung Study (Vestbo *et al.* 1999) used budesonide 800 µg/day (with 1.2 mg daily in the first six months of the Copenhagen study) – this is a little under 50 per cent of the equivalent dose used in Isolde. Lung Health-2 used triamcinolone 1.2 mg/day, which is about 20 per cent of the Isolde dosage. The meta-analysis made an attempt at dose response comparing a small number who received beclomethasone dipropionate 800 µg/day, with a larger number taking beclomethasone dipropionate 1500 µg/day or budesonide 1600 µg/day (van Grunsven *et al.* 1999). The 800 µg/day dosage had changes in FEV_1 indistinguishable from placebo, with improvement following the higher doses.

What are realistic outcome measures in the treatment of symptomatic COPD?

Most studies have used FEV_1 decline as the primary endpoint. Analysis of FEV_1 decline is difficult, particularly when dropouts are greater in those with the fastest FEV_1 decline, as is usual. The outcome is available for all severities, and is the most appropriate method for detecting early disease. Health-related quality of life is probably the best measure for moderate to severe disease. There is some question as to whether this method is sensitive enough in mild disease (the Copenhagen City Lung study used the Person General Wellbeing Scale which failed to detect abnormality in their group). Exacerbations are largely confined to those with more advanced disease, making it an important endpoint for this group. Exacerbations are the major health-care cost, and are particularly important in health economic studies. Mortality is an important outcome for those with severe disease. Measurement of gas transfer (D_{LCO}) is difficult to standardise sufficiently to make it a viable outcome measure. Emphysema is probably best tracked with serial CT scanning (Dirksen *et al.* 1997) but the methodology for emphysema quantification is not sufficiently widely available to make this a realistic outcome measure for large multicentre studies.

Survival

Increased survival is probably the only outcome that will convince the sceptics of effective treatments in severe COPD. Long-term oxygen therapy is the only widely accepted long-term treatment for COPD. It is not known to influence disease progression, symptoms or health-related quality of life (Heaton *et al.* 1993), but does prolong survival in hypoxic patients (Anonymous 1980, 1981). Mortality is only an appropriate outcome in end-stage disease and no prospective study has yet been completed with death as a primary outcome. Isolde showed a borderline significant survival advantage for the active group, with the survival lines diverging after nine months of therapy (Waterhouse *et al.* 1999). The Canadian observation study showed a significant 26 per cent reduction in mortality in those prescribed an inhaled corticosteroid in the months following discharge, compared with the group without such prescription (after adjusting for co-morbidity) (Sin & Tu 2001).

Health-related quality of life

It is unlikely that a study showing survival advantage in a chronic disabling disease would be accepted now unless the increased survival had some 'quality'. Advanced COPD limits the physical domains of questionnaires (for instance the SF36) much more than the mental and pain domains, which are relatively 'normal' (Spencer *et al.* 2001). It is unlikely to be a useful outcome in pre-symptomatic individuals. The Copenhagen City Lung Study found no impairment in health-related quality of life. Health-related quality of life deteriorates as the disease progresses. Responses to the St George's Respiratory Questionnaire (SGRQ), a disease-specific questionnaire, was a major outcome variable for Isolde, where it was measured every six months. The SGRQ scores deteriorated with time and the rate of deterioration was significantly reduced in the fluticasone group (Burge *et al.* 2000; Spencer *et al.* 2001). Significant differences were present in all three domains of the questionnaire, but were greatest for the symptom domain. The differences increased linearly over time. Similar differences were seen in the Weir study using the Guyatt questionnaire, although the differences were not statistically significant. Health-related quality of life was not studied in Euroscop. The SF36 was used in Lung Health-2, and showed no significant change (Lung Health Study Research Group 2000). The SF36 is a generic questionnaire and is less sensitive to change of respiratory disease than the disease-specific SGRQ and Guyatt questionnaires. Nevertheless there were significant improvements in the physical domains of the SF36 in the Isolde study. The differences between the outcomes of Isolde and Lung Health-2 could be due to differences in inhaled corticosteroid dosage (which the author believes is more likely), or to differences in disease severity. There is, however, a substantial overlap between the disease severity of patients recruited to both studies, and FEV_1 was not a determinant of SGRQ change in Isolde.

Symptoms

Symptom data is usually included within the health-related quality of life scores. The incidence of new symptoms was a specific outcome variable of Lung Health-2. There was a significant reduction in the onset or deterioration of cough, wheeze and difficulty breathing in the triamcinolone group.

Exacerbations

Health costs are dominated by the costs of managing exacerbations, particularly if these result in hospital admission. When total costs are measured, time off work with exacerbations is a dominant cost for more mild exacerbations. Health-related quality of life deteriorates with an exacerbation and is slow to recover. Exacerbations are more frequent as the disease progresses, making it a poor outcome for mild disease (there were very few exacerbations in the Copenhagen City Lung Study or Euroscop). Clinically defined exacerbations were specific outcomes for Isolde, the Exacerbation and the Weir studies, all of which showed reductions in exacerbation rates (Table 6.2). These rates are likely to be underestimates as those with the most frequent exacerbations were withdrawn (by design) from the studies. The meta-analysis reported the smallest reduction in exacerbations, the group taking beclomethasone 800 μg/day were included in the overall figures. The Canadian observation study showed a 23 per cent reduction in re-admissions in the group prescribed inhaled corticosteroids following first discharge (Sin & Tu 2001).

Table 6.2 Exacerbation rates (number/year) in the main studies referenced

	Isolde	Meta-analysis	Exacerbation	Weir	Euroscop	Copenhagen
Placebo	1.9	1.0	1.6**	0.57	3.1*	0.38
Inhaled steroid	1.43	0.9	1.07**	0.36	2.2*	0.36
Reduction (%)	25	10	49	37	29	2

*   percentage taking at least one course of prednisolone during the trial for COPD exacerbation
**   total exacerbations/year

Lung function

The rate of decline in FEV_1 was the primary endpoint in the design of all the longer studies. None showed a statistically convincing change in the rate of decline. This was unexpected in light of the substantial effects seen in the smaller and shorter-term studies where FEV_1 decline was generally calculated from the difference between the first and last readings, or linear modelling through the baseline data point (Table 6.3). The larger studies allowed more complex mixed effects modelling which may be less powerful in differentiating treatment effects. The model used for the Isolde analysis allowed the regression line to be independent of the baseline value, to model the initial increase in FEV_1 better. The greater the initial effect, the greater the subsequent slope. The Copenhagen City Lung study showed absolutely no treatment effect on FEV_1 decline, nor did it show an initial improvement in the FEV_1 (Table 6.4). The study convincingly shows that budesonide 800 μg/day was without effect in this group with the most mild disease. Euroscop showed a small initial effect

Table 6.3 FEV$_1$ decline from the shorter studies mostly using linear modelling from baseline measurements

	Meta-analysis 800 µg/day	1500–1600 µg/day	Exacerbation	Weir
Placebo	0	0	0	−45.2
Inhaled steroid	+2	+39	+80 (6 months)	−12.1

Table 6.4 Modelled FEV$_1$ for the three-year studies; initial effect in ml (compared with placebo), subsequent decline in millilitres/year (the figure for the initial change in FEV$_1$ is an approximation for the Euroscop study due to different methodology)

	Isolde		Euroscop		Copenhagen		Lung Health-2	
	Initial (ml)	Decline (ml/year)	Initial (ml)	Decline (ml/year)	Initial (ml)	Decline (ml/year)	Initial (ml)	Decline (ml/year)
Placebo	0	−59	0	−69	0	49.6	0	47.0
Inhaled steroid	+55	−50	+8.5	−57	0	53.2	0	44.2
Reduction		9		12		3.6		2.8

with a 12 ml/year difference in the slopes of FEV$_1$ decline between budesonide and placebo. The slopes were significantly different (for the group who had smoked the least) when the population was divided into two groups based on pack-years smoked, the supposition being that those who were the most susceptible to smoking, who had reached the same lower level of FEV$_1$ with less smoking, were the ones with the greatest benefit. Isolde showed the largest initial effect, which was significantly greater in the ex-smokers compared with the current smokers. The subsequent decline in FEV$_1$ was 9 ml/year less in the fluticasone group. The effect of fluticasone on subsequent FEV$_1$ decline was additive to the effects of continued smoking during the trial, and independent of the effect of a two-week oral steroid trial which followed randomisation.

There are unexplained differences between the estimates of FEV$_1$ decline using these models and those observed using linear regression before study entry. For instance the Euroscop study had a six-month run-in with no active treatment (in individuals who had not previously taken inhaled steroids). The mean FEV$_1$ declined 113 ml/year in those subsequently randomised to placebo. The mixed effects model for the three years on placebo gave an estimate of 69 ml/year. Similar figures for the Isolde study where the run-in was only two months were 220 ml/year during the run-in (steroid naïve subgroup) and 59 ml/year for the modelled three-year placebo group. The Copenhagen City Lung Study had a measurement of FEV$_1$ 13 years previously in the majority of their subjects. The rates of decline during these 13 years and during the placebo three-year treatment were similar at 52 and 49.6 ml/year respectively. These differences are worrying: they could be due to the positive effect of taking part in a trial with enhanced expectations and better treatment of exacerbations in those randomised to placebo, or could be due to a failure of the mixed effects models to incorporate the data adequately from rapid decliners who withdraw before the end of the study. In either case it makes it difficult to show significant changes in FEV_1 decline over a three- to five-year study. No significant effects have been seen (using an intention to treat analysis and a mixed effects model or similar) with any randomised intervention including smoking cessation (Anthonisen *et al.* 1994; Vestbo *et al.* 1999; Burge *et al.* 2000). Several studies have also been hampered by an initial improvement in FEV_1 of 8–100 ml. This is a clinically insignificant change, but in terms of a 30 ml/year annual decline it is large, and usually precludes using all the data in the model, which has to be confined to the period after any short-term effect has stabilised (Anthonisen *et al.* 1994; Pauwels *et al.* 1999; Burge *et al.* 2000).

Treatment toxicity

Studies of long-term oral corticosteroids have showed major toxicity limiting their use (Postma *et al.* 1985). Euroscop specifically investigated fractures and showed no increase in fractures in the budesonide group. A substudy measured bone density longitudinally, the only statistical difference being for greater trochanter bone density which was better in the budesonide group (Pauwels *et al.* 1999). The lack of effect may depend on the corticosteroid used, as Lung Health-2 did show increased bone loss in the triamcinolone group (Lung Health Study Research Group 2000). There was no increase in cataracts over this short period of time (Pauwels *et al.* 1999; Burge *et al.* 2000). Inhaled corticosteroids are associated with bruising, probably due to skin thinning, Euroscop counted arm bruises at each visit, the budesonide group has a cumulative incidence of 10 per cent compared with 4 per cent for those taking placebo. Isolde and Euroscop both showed increases in oral *Candida* and in throat irritation, in line with studies of these drugs in asthma. Serum cortisol levels were 20–30 nmol/l lower in the budesonide and fluticasone groups compared with placebo. This compares with a reduction of 220 nmol/l with the addition of 5 mg prednisolone in one small study (Renkema *et al.* 1996).

Economic outcomes

There are a few studies estimating the medical costs of treatment, using relatively simple models with drug costs, doctor visits (emergency and routine) and hospital admissions. In the Exacerbation study fluticasone 1 mg/day was cost neutral (Hurrell *et al.* 1999). In patients not selected for exacerbation rate treatment may cost more than no treatment, but there is an advantage in terms of symptoms, health-related quality of life and lung function. There are no established parameters with which to compare drug costs in this group.

Who should (or should not) receive inhaled steroids, and at what dose?

Existing treatment is not going to repair the alveolar walls lost in emphysema or refashion the fibrosed bronchioles in obstructive bronchitis, so realistic outcomes of treatment are required. The Isolde study clearly shows benefit in terms of reduced exacerbations and better health-related quality of life in the fluticasone group (as well as higher levels of FEV_1); all the measured differences between fluticasone and placebo increased throughout the three years of the trial. These effects are supported by the other studies in moderate to severe disease, and by the Canadian observation study. Withdrawal of inhaled steroids in this group results in an unacceptably high incidence of exacerbations (Jarad *et al.* 1999). Patients with moderate to severe disease are more likely to be helped than damaged by high doses of inhaled steroids. Some might want to limit the use of inhaled steroids in this group. They are warranted in those with at least yearly exacerbations, those with symptoms and those with accelerated loss of FEV_1. Response cannot be predicted by smoking status, atopy or response to a short course of oral steroids. The Copenhagen study clearly shows no benefit in those with the mildest disease and no impairment of health-related quality of life. Few in this group are likely to develop disabling COPD. The problem arises with the intermediate group who have few symptoms and relatively well-preserved levels of FEV_1. As treatment in endstage disease slows rather than reverses disease progression, earlier treatment is required. Here the efficacy of inhaled corticosteroids remains to be proven. Euroscop addressed this most important group, but is, unfortunately, the unexpected early increase in FEV_1 limited the power of the study using FEV_1 as an outcome, and the lack of a health-related quality-of-life measure removed this as a measurable outcome. Lung Health-2 studied an important intermediate group but used a very low dose of a non-selective corticosteroid; there was some benefit in terms of reduced new symptoms. The author believes that those with more mild disease with measured rapid decline in FEV_1 or frequent exacerbations warrant treatment (Isolde included patients with an FEV_1 up to 85 per cent predicted).

There is little data on dose–response. The studies with the greatest benefit have used at least 1.5 mg beclomethasone, 1.6 mg budesonide or 1 mg fluticasone daily. The meta-analysis has a small group with beclomethasone 800 µg/day, who did no better than placebo. On current evidence high doses are required. Toxicity is a manageable problem. Oral symptoms are similar to those seen in asthmatics, bruising is common in elderly smokers and does not usually excite much attention in the absence of steroid therapy, the evidence on bone loss in this group is reassuring (with the exception of those taking triamcinolone). The author hopes there will be better and more specific treatments than inhaled steroids in the future, but at present the risk–benefit ratio clearly favours high-dose inhaled steroids in this disabled and neglected group of patients.

Recommendations

Inhaled corticosteroids reduce exacerbations, and reduce the decline in health-related quality of life compared with placebo. They are warranted in patients with regular exacerbations and significant symptoms. The higher levels of FEV_1 following inhaled corticosteroid treatment are modest and unlikely to be the sole reason for prescribing these drugs. There is no evidence of treatment advantage between beclomethasone 1.5–2 mg, budesonide 1.6 mg and fluticasone 1 mg daily, the doses for which benefit has been shown. Lower-dose triamcinolone appears to cause more bone demineralisation and has no specific advantages to recommend its use. The place for inhaled corticosteroid treatment in pre-symptomatic disease remains to be established.

References

Anonymous (1980). Continuous or nocturnal oxygen therapy in hypoxemic chronic obstructive lung disease: a clinical trial. Nocturnal Oxygen Therapy Trial Group. *Annals of Internal Medicine* **93**, 391–398

Anonymous (1981). Long term domiciliary oxygen therapy in chronic hypoxic cor pulmonale complicating chronic bronchitis and emphysema. Report of the Medical Research Council Working Party. *Lancet* **1**, 681–686

Anthonisen NR, Connett JE, Kiley JP *et al.* (1994) Effects of smoking intervention and the use of an inhaled anticholinergic bronchodilator on the rate of decline of FEV1. The Lung Health Study. *Journal of the American Medical Association* **272**, 1497–1505

Burge PS, Calverley PMA, Jones PW, Spencer SA, Anderson JA, Maslen TK (2000). Randomised, double blind, placebo controlled study of fluticasone propionate in patients with moderate to severe chronic obstructive pulmonary disease; the ISOLDE trial. *British Medical Journal* **320**, 1297–1303

Dirksen A, Friis M, Olesen KP, Skovgaard LT, Sorensen K (1997). Progress of emphysema in severe alpha-1-antitrypsin deficiency as assessed by annual CT. *Acta Radiologica* **38**, 826–832

Heaton RK, Grant I, McSweeny AJ, Adams KM, Petty TL (1983). Psychologic effects of continuous and nocturnal oxygen therapy in hypoxemic chronic obstructive pulmonary disease. *Archives of Internal Medicine* **143**, 1941–1947

Hurrell C, Price M, Hollingworth K, Thwaites R (1999). Cost effectiveness of inhaled fluticasone propionate in the treatment of patients with chronic obstructive pulmonary disease (COPD). *American Journal of Respiratory & Critical Care Medicine* **159**, A797

Jarad NA, Wedzicha JA, Burge PS *et al.* (1999). An observational study of inhaled corticosteroid withdrawal in stable chronic obstructive pulmonary disease. *Respiratory Medicine* **93**, 161–166

Lung Health Study Research Group (2000). Effects of inhaled triamcinolone on the decline in pulmonary function in chronic obstructive pulmonary disease. *New England Journal of Medicine* **343**, 1902–1909

Paggiaro PL, Dahle R, Bakran I, Frith L, Hollingworth K, Efthimiou J (1998). Multicentre randomised placebo-controlled trial of inhaled fluticasone propionate in patients with chronic obstructive pulmonary disease. International COPD Study Group. *Lancet* **351**, 773–780

Pauwels RA, Lofdahl C, Laitinen LA *et al.* (1999). Long-term treatment with inhaled budesonide in persons with mild chronic obstructive pulmonary disease who continue smoking. *New England Journal of Medicine* **340**, 1948–1953

Postma DS, Steenhuis EJ, Van de Weele LT, Sluiter HJ (1985). Severe chronic airflow obstruction. Can corticosteroids slow down progression? *European Journal of Respiratory Disease* **67**, 56–64

Renkema TE, Schouten JP, Koeter GH, Postma DS (1996). Effects of long-term treatment with corticosteroids in COPD. *Chest* **109**, 1156–1162

Sin DD & Tu JV (2001). Impact of inhaled steroids in elderly patients with chronic obstructive pulmonary disease. *American Journal of Respiratory Critical Care Medicine* **161**, A490

Spencer S, Calverley PMA, Burge PS, Jones PW (2001). Health status deterioration in patients with chronic obstructive pulmonary disease. *American Journal of Respiratory & Critical Care Medicine* **163**, 122–128

van Grunsven PM, van Schayck CP, Derenne JP *et al.* (1999). Long term effects of inhaled corticosteroids in chronic obstructive pulmonary disease: a meta-analysis. *Thorax* **54**, 7–14

Vestbo J, Sorensen T, Lange P, Brix A, Torre P, Viskum K (1999). Long-term effects of inhaled budesonide in mild and moderate chronic obstructive pulmonary disease: a randomised controlled trial. *Lancet* **353**, 1819–1823

Waterhouse JC, Fishwick D, Anderson JA, Calverley PMA, Burge PS (1999). What caused death in the Isolde study. *European Respiratory Journal* **14**, 387s

Weir DC, Weiland GA, Burge PS *et al.* (1994). Decline in FEV1 in patients with chronic airflow obstruction. Relation to acute steroid response and treatment with inhaled corticosteroids. In Postma DS & Gerritsen J (eds) *Bronchitis V*. Assen: Van Gorcum, pp280–286

Weir DC, Bale GA, Bright P, Burge PS (1999). A double-blind placebo-controlled study of the effect of inhaled beclomethasone dipropionate for 2 years in patients with nonasthmatic chronic obstructive pulmonary disease. *Clinical and Experimental Allergy* **29**, 125–128

Chapter 7

Scientific evidence and expert clinical opinion for the selection and use of novel therapies: clinical decision making in individual cases

Elizabeth E Gamble and Neil C Barnes

Introduction

Considering drug treatment choices in the future, one needs to consider the main problems in chronic obstructive pulmonary disease (COPD): the heterogeneity of the disease and the clinical effectiveness of currently available therapies. The main problems in COPD are the continuing symptoms of shortness of breath, the risk of exacerbations of the disease and the increased mortality (American Thoracic Society 1995). The risk of mortality is related to the impairment in lung function as measured by the forced expiratory volume in 1 second (FEV_1) (Anthonisen *et al.* 1986). The only therapeutic manoeuvres, which have been shown to have a major effect on mortality, are cessation of smoking (Anthonisen *et al.* 1994) and oxygen therapy in hypoxic patients with cor pulmonale (Nocturnal Oxygen Therapy Trial Group 1980; Medical Research Council Working Party 1981). Smoking cessation slows the accelerated decline in FEV_1 and therefore decreases mortality and decreases the risk of disease exacerbation. Other therapies have not been shown to decrease mortality, although they may have a small but, in the context of the disease, clinically useful effect on symptoms and disease exacerbations. Long-acting β_2 agonists and anticholinergic drugs produce improvements in symptoms (O'Donnell *et al.* 1999; Lotvall 2000) and there is the theoretical possibility that long-acting β_2 agonists may have a beneficial effect on exacerbations of COPD (Kips 2000). Inhaled steroids decrease exacerbations of COPD in patients with more severe disease, but the effect on pulmonary function and symptoms is at best modest (Burge *et al.* 2000).

Pathology

Against this background, any drug that had a beneficial effect on symptoms, preventing exacerbations or slowing the rate of decline of FEV_1 and therefore the risk of mortality, would be of benefit. There are several problems associated with developing a drug that would have such a beneficial impact. It is now clear from a number of studies that, in patients with COPD but no features of asthma, the inflammatory profile is quite distinct from that of asthma. In asthma there is an increase in CD4+ T cells, eosinophils and thickening of the basement membrane with epithelial disruption (Bousquet *et al.* 2000). In contrast, in COPD there is an increase in CD8+ T cells, macrophages (O'Shaughnessy *et al.* 1997) and in severe disease neutrophils (Di Stefano *et al.* 1998). Epithelial disruption is not typical, but there may be squamous metaplasia. Basement membrane thickness is within the normal range (Jeffery 2000). Two studies have demonstrated an association between the number of CD8+ T cells and disease severity (O'Shaughnessy *et al.* 1997; Lams *et al.* 2000). There have been preliminary reports of studies investigating the effect of inhaled corticosteroids on the inflammatory profile of COPD (Hattotuwa *et al.* 1999, 2000). It is clear that, while there are effects on the immunopathology, these fall far short of those seen in asthma. It is therefore likely that one important approach to new drug development will be the discovery of a drug that beneficially impacts on the specific inflammatory profile in COPD.

Heterogeneity of COPD

One factor that will have to be considered in relation to this is that clearly COPD is a heterogeneous condition. It has generally been considered that the clinical picture of COPD can be caused by a variable combination of three distinct pathological processes. These are the alveolar destruction of emphysema, mucous gland hypertrophy and inflammation of chronic bronchitis, and late-onset and largely irreversible asthma. Most of the biopsy studies that have been performed so far in COPD have investigated a group of patients with no features suggestive of asthma and found the increase in CD8+ T cells, increased macrophages, no thickening of the basement membrane and no evidence of epithelial disruption as mentioned above. One study has investigated a mixed group of patients (Chanez *et al.* 1997). Biopsies were performed in a group of patients with clinical COPD and they were then given a standard trial with oral corticosteroids. Only those patients with evidence of increased eosinophils in bronchoalveolar lavage and thickening of the reticular basement membrane improved with corticosteroids. It is possible, therefore, that some drugs may only be active in a subset of patients. Clinical trials and subsequent clinical usage of the drug in this circumstance may require a combination of a diagnostic test to determine the subgroup and the targeted therapy.

Most of the focus in developing new drugs for COPD has been on impacting directly on the lung disease, but other aspects of the disease need to be considered. Many patients become socially isolated and depressed and effective antidepressants for this group would be of immense value. Many patients, particularly with more severe disease and emphysema, become cachectic and malnourished. Treatment of these dietary problems has proved difficult and effective strategies for dealing with this problem would also be of value.

Conclusion

In conclusion, any new drug that beneficially affected the three main problems in COPD, namely symptoms, exacerbations and the accelerated decline in lung function leading to an increased mortality, would be of clinical benefit. It is likely that some drugs may only be of value in particular subsets of patients. Of the new drugs currently being investigated, promise is being shown with phosphodiesterase type 4 isoenzyme inhibitors which in early clinical trials seem to show benefit in terms of improvement in pulmonary function, symptoms and exercise capacity (Compton *et al.* 1999a, 1999b).

References

American Thoracic Society (1995). Standards for the diagnosis and care of patients with chronic obstructive pulmonary disease. *American Journal of Respiratory & Critical Care Medicine* **152**, S77–S120

Anthonisen NR, Connett JE, Kiley JP *et al.* (1994). Effects of smoking intervention and the use of inhaled anticholinergic bronchodilator on the rate of decline of FEV_1. The Lung Health Study. *Journal of the American Medical Association* **272**, 1497–1505

Anthonisen NR, Wright EC, Hodgkin JE (1986). Prognosis in chronic obstructive pulmonary disease. *American Review of Respiratory Disease* **133**, 14–20

Bousquet J, Jeffery PK, Busse WW, Johnson M, Vignola AM (2000). Asthma. From bronchoconstriction to airways inflammation and remodeling. *American Journal of Respiratory & Critical Care Medicine* **161**, 1720–1745

Burge PS, Calverley PM, Jones PW, Spencer S, Anderson JA, Maslen TK (2000). Randomised, double blind, placebo controlled study of fluticasone propionate in patients with moderate to severe chronic obstructive pulmonary disease: the ISOLDE trial. *British Medical Journal* **320**, 1297–1303

Chanez P, Vignola AM, O'Shaughnessy T *et al.* (1997). Corticosteroid reversibility in COPD is related to features of asthma. *American Journal of Respiratory & Critical Care Medicine* **155**, 1529–1534

Compton CH, Gubb J, Cedar E *et al.* (1999a). Ariflo (SB 207499), a second generation, oral PDE4 inhibitor, improves quality of life in patients with COPD [Abstract]. *American Journal of Respiratory & Critical Care Medicine* **159**, A522

Compton CH, Gubb J, Cedar E *et al.* (1999b). The efficacy of Ariflo (SB 207499), a second generation, oral PDE4 inhibitor, in patients with COPD [Abstract]. *American Journal of Respiratory & Critical Care Medicine* **159**, A806

Di Stefano A, Capelli A, Lusuardi M *et al.* (1998). Severity of airflow limitation is associated with severity of airway inflammation in smokers. *American Journal of Respiratory & Critical Care Medicine* **158**, 1277–1285

Hattotuwa K, Ansari T, Gizycki M, Barnes N, Jeffery PK (1999). A double blind placebo-controlled trial of the effect of inhaled corticosteroids on the immunopathology of COPD. *American Journal of Respiratory & Critical Care Medicine* **159**, A523

Hattotuwa K, Matin D, Ansari TW, Gizycki MJ, Jeffery PK (2000). Inhaled steroids decreases mast cells in moderate to severe COPD [Abstract]. *American Journal of Respiratory & Critical Care Medicine* **161**, A491

Jeffery PK (2000). Comparison of the structural and inflammatory features of COPD and asthma (Giles F. Filley Lecture). *Chest* **117**, 251s–260s

Kips J (2000). The clinical role of long-acting beta2-agonists in COPD. *Respiratory Medicine* **94**, S1–S5

Lams BE, Sousa AR, Rees PJ, Lee TH (2000). Subepithelial immunopathology of large airways in smokers with and without chronic obstructive pulmonary disease. *European Respiratory Journal* **15**, 512–516

Lotvall J (2000). Pharmacology of bronchodilators used in the treatment of COPD. *Respiratory Medicine* **94**, S6–S10

Medical Research Council Working Party (1981). Long term domiciliary oxygen therapy in chronic hypoxic cor pulmonale complicating chronic bronchitis and emphysema. *Lancet* **i**, 681–686

Nocturnal Oxygen Therapy Trial Group (1980). Continuous or nocturnal oxygen therapy in hypoxaemic chronic obstructive lung disease. *Annals of Internal Medicine* **93**, 391–398

O'Donnell DE, Lam M, Webb KA (1999). Spirometric correlates of improvement in exercise performance after anticholinergic therapy in chronic obstructive pulmonary disease. *American Journal of Respiratory & Critical Care Medicine* **160**, 542–549

O'Shaughnessy T, Ansari TW, Barnes NC, Jeffery PK (1997). Inflammation in bronchial biopsies of subjects with chronic bronchitis: inverse relationship of CD8[+] T lymphocytes with FEV_1. *American Journal of Respiratory & Critical Care Medicine* **155**, 852–857

PART 3

Evidence and opinion for surgical intervention

Chapter 8

Lung volume reduction surgery and lung transplantation for COPD

John H Dark

Introduction

Surgery has, until recently, had a small role in the management of emphysema, limited to dealing with intrapleural complications and occasional resections for bullous disease. For carefully selected patients with more severe forms of chronic obstructive pulmonary disease (COPD) indications and outcomes in lung transplantation are now well defined. There remain important debates about organ allocation for different diagnostic groups and, within emphysema patients, between the merits of single and bilateral lung transplantation.

On the other hand, lung volume reduction surgery, particularly in the UK, does not yet have a defined role. There are major debates over patient selection and even type of procedure. Long-term outcome is largely unknown although it is accepted that most patients will deteriorate back to their baseline status over the course of a few years. A number of randomised, prospective, controlled trials have demonstrated a short and medium advantage compared with pulmonary rehabilitation alone. However, the really important and unresolved questions have yet to be subjected to scientific study.

Historical background

Brantigan *et al.* (1957) are widely credited as being the first to describe the reduction of lung volume by surgical means as a treatment for patients with emphysema. This series, in the 1950s, was ill characterised and he abandoned the technique because of high peri-operative mortality. There had previously been a number of other mechanical approaches to the chest wall dysfunction. These have been described in detail and placed in an appropriate perspective (Gaensler *et al.* 1983; Deslauriers 1996).

In the modern era Cooper *et al.* (1995) was the first to describe lung volume reduction surgery (LVRS). In 20 highly selected patients they could demonstrate an 82 per cent improvement in forced expiratory volume in 1 second (FEV_1) with no operative mortality. A year later they had a series of 150 patients (Cooper *et al.* 1996) and several other groups were also publishing their experience. Laser bullectomy, a technique briefly popular in the western USA, was clearly shown to be inferior (McKenna *et al.* 1996b). The subsequent debates centred on whether the procedure should be unilateral or bilateral or whether it should be by an open or thoracoscopic (VAT) approach. There has been extensive, and as yet inconclusive, debate about patient selection (see below). On a wider scale, there remains debate about the overall costs and benefits on both sides of the Atlantic (Cranshaw & Evans 2001).

Clinical success in pulmonary transplantation was achieved in 1981 with heart–lung transplantation (Reitz *et al.* 1982) and 1985 for the single lung transplantation (Cooper *et al.* 1987). It was initially felt that a paired, i.e., a heart, lung or bilateral lung, transplantation would be required for emphysema. A number of patients had died during the 1970s because of gross overinflation of the native lung (Stevens *et al.* 1970). However, Mal *et al.* (1989) showed the single lung transplantation was entirely feasible for obstructive airways disease. Emphysema has now become the most common indication for this procedure throughout the world.

The alternative bilateral lung transplantation can also be applied to patients with emphysema. It may have a lower early mortality and in registry studies has an improved survival from between three and five years. These are, however, non-randomised patients and there has been a tendency to select the bilateral lung procedure for young fitter patients, leaving the more straightforward single lung transplantation for older patients. There does, however, seem to be a survival advantage if not an important functional difference in favour of the bilateral lung transplantation. This relatively wasteful use of scarce donor organs is difficult to reconcile with the data which suggests that emphysema patients, of all those undergoing lung transplantation, have least to gain in terms of improved life expectancy. There is a paradox in carrying out the relatively wasteful bilateral lung transplant procedure in a situation where most patients gain quality rather than quantity of life.

LVRS: indications, patient selection

LVRS is only applicable to a minority of patients with emphysema. Selection involves identification of appropriate physiology, exclusion of contraindications, and alternative options for treatment and, finally, balancing risk against the likely benefits.

The key attributes of patients selected is that they are overinflated (TLC >120 per cent of predicted) and have heterogeneous disease. The latter is identified by CT and isotope perfusion scanning. In general, areas of absent or reduced perfusion will correlate with areas of greatest parenchymal destruction (Figures 8.1 and 8.2) and these comprise target areas for resection. Whilst good results can clearly be obtained in patients with diffuse disease, the best results in terms of both early improvement and survival, are found in those with target areas, particularly at the apex of the lung (Hamacher *et al.* 1999).

A set of suggested indications and contraindications is set out in Tables 8.1 and 8.2. In general, FEV_1 will be less than 30–40 per cent of predicted – patients better than this should not be severely limited by emphysema. Even though they may have an improvement on spirometry, it does not justify the risk of surgery for this group.

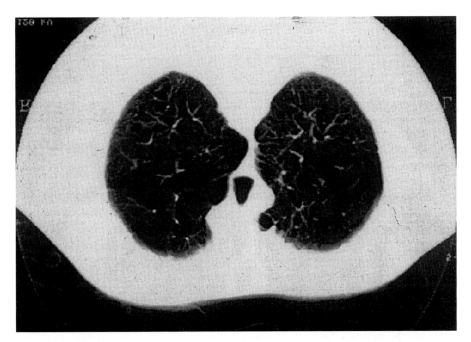

Figure 8.1 CT scan demonstrating severe, destructive emphysema at the lung apices

Table 8.1 Indications for LVRS

Disabled, despite full medical Rx
FEV_1 <40% predicted
TLC >120% predicted
(RV >200% predicted)
Hyperinflation, flattened diaphragm on chest x-ray
Target areas on CT, confirmed on isotope perfusion scan

Table 8.2 Contraindications to LVRS

Age >75–80
Other severe co-morbidity, e.g., coronary artery disease, obesity, cachexia, previous
thoracic surgery, pleurodesis (consider for unilateral procedure)
No hyperinflation – on chest x-ray
TLC <100% predicted, RV <150% predicted
Six-minute walk <150 metres
PCO_2 >6 kPa
Pulmonary artery systolic pressure >45 mmHg
Absence of target areas on CT scan or isotope perfusion scan
α_1-Antitrypsin deficiency

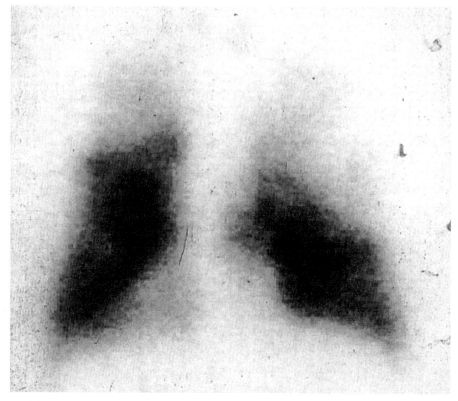

Figure 8.2 Isotope perfusion scan confirming apical target areas

Some patients are too severely affected, i.e., they do not have enough worthwhile lung to benefit from the mechanical improvement they receive. Their operative risks are very high. Hypercapnia (P_{CO_2} >6 kPa), pulmonary hypertension (pulmonary artery systolic pressure >45 mmHg) and severely impaired gas transfer (D_{LCO} <30 per cent of predicted) are all markers of high risk, poor outcome and are contraindications. Poor rehabilitation, or an inability to rehabilitate, is another contraindication and a minimum six-minute walk distance of 150 metres is suggested (Geddes *et al.* 2000). In practice, selection of very well-motivated patients with ideal physiology who have undergone extended rehabilitation, will tend to give the best results. Such an approach probably explains the strikingly low mortality rate in several North American series (Cooper *et al.* 1996; Keenan *et al.* 1996; Naunheim *et al.* 1996). Standard investigations are listed in Table 8.3.

Patients who are turned down for lung transplantation because of co-morbidities such as osteoporosis, inability to wean off steroids or impaired cardiac function, are also high-risk candidates for LVRS.

Table 8.3 Assessment for LVRS – investigations

Spirometry
Lung volumes (by whole body plethysmography)
Arterial blood gases
Chest x-ray and CT scan
Isotope perfusion scan
Cardiac echo
Six-minute walk or shuttle test

Surgical approach

The classic procedure is bilateral LVRS via a sternotomy. The patient is anaesthetised after placement of a thoracic epidural then has a double-lumen endotracheal tube. Arterial monitoring of blood pressure is essential. Air trapping with subsequent haemodynamic collapse (treated by opening the endotracheal tube to air) may easily occur after starting mechanical ventilation. Pulse oximetry and monitoring of end-tidal CO_2 are clearly essential. Patients should be extubated and breathing spontaneously at the end of the procedure, but nevertheless should be nursed in an ITU for at least the first 12–24 hours.

After sternotomy, opening of the pleural spaces and division of all adhesions between the lung and the chest wall, one lung anaesthesia is commenced. Poorly perfused areas of the non-ventilated lung will remain inflated, and are the target areas. This visual examination correlates well with the CT scan and isotope perfusion scan. These portions of lung, typically at the apex, are removed by repeated application of mechanical staplers. Reinforcement with strips of pericardium reduces air leak (Miller *et al.* 1996). The deflated lung should be carefully palpated for nodules. Up to 15 per cent of patients had T1 lung cancers found by chance either on pre-operative CT scan or in the resected specimen (Ojo *et al.* 1997). The reinflated lung should be checked meticulously for air leaks. Time spent ensuring an intact lung is repaid in the shorter post-operative stay.

In the post-operative phase no suction should be applied to drains even if there is a pneumothorax. Patients are often hypercapnic for a few hours and the lung will usually become fully inflated in a non-traumatic fashion by normal inspiration. Prolonged air leak, despite all these precautions, is common. Heimlich valves, rather than underwater sealed drains, allow early mobilisation. The author has used a mini-tracheostomy placed through the crico-thyroid membrane at any suggestion of sputum retention or poor clearance of secretions.

Standard lateral thoracotomy is not widely used and the principal debate is between open (sternotomy) and VAT approaches. There are no randomised trials, and comparisons of apparently matched patients have produced conflicting results. Retrospective studies suggest a similar mortality, equally good function outcome but longer ITU stay, more complications and more respiratory failure in the sternotomy group (Wisser *et al.* 1997; Hazelrigg *et al.* 1998). Only one study had a higher mortality for sternotomy (Kotloff *et al.* 1996). These reports all have a historical bias with VAT procedures performed more recently.

Bilateral procedures have a better functional outcome than unilateral – 57 per cent versus 31 per cent improvement in FEV$_1$ at six months in one study (McKenna *et al.* 1996a). The same patients also had improved one-year survival rate – 95 per cent versus 83 per cent. There seems to be no advantage for a unilateral approach unless previous surgery – pleurodesis for instance – prevents safe entry into a pleural space, or if there is asymmetrical disease with only target areas in one lung. A few patients have had combined LVRS and lung resection for tumour with excellent results – both low mortality and functional improvement and these procedures are clearly unilateral.

Laser shrinkage, popularised by Wakabayashi (1995), has been subject to a randomised control trial and is clearly inferior to staple resection (McKenna *et al.* 1996b).

Outcomes of LVRS

Pulmonary function

The initial report of Cooper *et al.* (1995) documented an 82 per cent improvement in FEV$_1$ six months after bilateral LVRS via sternotomy. This series, of scrupulously selected and thoroughly rehabilitated patients, has rarely been bettered. In a review article, improvements ranging from 13–96 per cent were recorded (Flaherty & Fernando 2000). However, a collected review published in *Thorax* (Young *et al.* 1999) found only an overall increase in FEV$_1$ of 220 ml in 925 patients. FEV$_1$ has been used as a principal endpoint in these studies and there is no doubt that the majority of patients will make gains, often very significant gains. It nevertheless remains a feature of LVRS that a proportion of patients, probably never less than 10 per cent, gain little improvement.

There are no important differences between open and VAT approaches (Wisser *et al.* 1977; Kotloff *et al.* 1996): unilateral LVRS consistently gives less good improvement. In all major series a proportion, typically a fifth but up to 50 per cent, have less than a 20 per cent improvement in FEV$_1$. Some of these patients are poorly selected, probably with diffuse disease and no obvious target areas. Some had α_1-antitrypsin deficiency, now known to be a group who do badly (Cassina *et al.* 1998; Gelb *et al.* 1999). Nevertheless, it remains a feature of LVRS that a proportion of patients, probably never less than 10 per cent, gained little improvement.

There are at least three published randomised controlled trials comparing LVRS and exercise rehabilitation alone. Criner *et al.* (1999) randomised 37 patients and found significantly improved FEV$_1$ in the LVRS arm. There were no deaths in this study in either arm. Both LVRS and rehabilitation improved six-minute walk and dyspnoea score but the objective improvements in pulmonary function were only found in the surgical arm. In the UK, Geddes *et al.* (2000) randomised 48 patients,

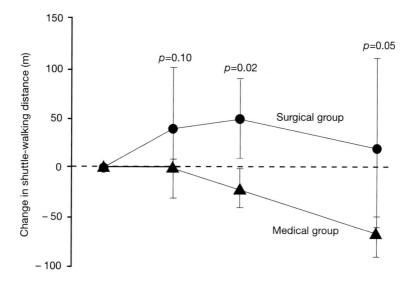

Figure 8.3 Short-term improvement in patients randomised to LVRS, compared with pulmonary rehabilitation. Subsequently the surgical group deteriorate at the same rate as the controls. From Geddes *et al.* (2000)

24 to continued rehabilitation and 24 to surgery. There were more deaths in the surgical arm (five versus three) and an improved FEV_1 of only 70 ml. The medical group lost an average of 80 ml of FEV_1 in the same time period (Figure 8.3). Those undergoing LVRS subsequently had a progressive fall in FEV_1 at the same rate as the medical group. Heterogeneous disease was not a criterion for acceptance into this study, perhaps explaining the disappointing results. In contrast, 60 patients were randomised by a group in Rome (Pompeo *et al.* 2000). They had heterogeneous disease, on CT, as a primary entry criterion. At both three and six months post-op there was a mean improvement of 53 per cent in FEV_1, amounting to 460 ml. Again those randomised to rehabilitation showed improvement in exercise capacity and dyspnoea score but no change in FEV_1.

Most papers report improvements in six-minute walk distance and various measures of dyspnoea score, in parallel with FEV_1. As would be expected, TLC and RV consistently fall, typically by 20–30 per cent, or approximately 2 litres.

Many reports, particularly from American centres, also document a reduced proportion of patients requiring supplemental oxygen and an increased number weaned off steroids. The latter is difficult to explain, given that the great bulk of these patients should have steroid-unresponsive airway obstruction.

Mortality and morbidity

Adverse events after surgery largely relate to the degree of patient selection. Mortality rates of between 0 and 19 per cent have been recorded (Young *et al.* 1999) and an informal review of UK experience suggested a mortality rate of between 12 and 17 per cent. It did, however, represent preliminary experience at many centres.

As would be expected in any surgical procedure on patients with borderline respiratory function, there is an incidence of respiratory failure and need for a tracheostomy. Persistent air leak can be measured by standard techniques including Heimlich valves and many of these problems can be treated on an outpatient basis. The change in mortality in the randomised study reported by Geddes *et al.* (2000), when entry criteria were tightened, is a good example of the influence of patient selection on post-surgical outcome. There is little useful data on long-term survival. Patients taken on for surgery clearly are a selected group, with other co-morbidities excluded, and they cannot be readily compared with non-surgical patients. The numbers were too small in the randomised controlled trials although intuitively one would expect an increase in FEV_1 to be mirrored by an increase in survival. In one study, patients with the greatest short-lived improvement in FEV_1 had the best long-term survival (Brenner *et al.* 1999). There is one report of a group of 22 patients, accepted for LVRS, who were denied surgery because of a change in Medicare funding. Thirty six per cent of them died compared with the 17 per cent of age- and function-matched patients who underwent surgery in the same time scale (Meyers *et al.* 1998).

Long-term results

It would be fair to say that there is no good long-term data about survival after LVRS. There is accumulating data to demonstrate that the rate of loss of lung function remains similar to that experienced by patients with emphysema as a whole. This is particularly well illustrated in Figure 8.3 taken from the report from Geddes *et al.* (2000). It has been suggested that there is a symptomatic benefit even when FEV_1 has returned to baseline levels. Such patients will often still have a residual volume lower than pre-operatively. They clearly have the advantage of increased exercise capacity and possibly improved appetite during the post-surgical phase which leads to a better quality of life even when spirometry has reduced again.

Lung transplantation: selection of recipients

In general, transplantation should be offered to patients who have advanced lung disease for whom all alternative treatments have been exhausted and for whom life expectancy is no more than 2–3 years. For COPD patients, the indications are set down in Table 8.4. Patients have to be suitable for rehabilitation: those who are severely debilitated or bed bound will have a difficult and high-risk post-operative course.

Table 8.4 Broad indications for lung transplantation in COPD

$FEV_1 < 25\%$ predicted after bronchodilator therapy
Significant hypoxia (oxygen dependent) and/or hypocapnia rapid decline in lung function
Frequent exacerbations requiring hospital admission: episodes of assisted ventilation

In general, patients with COPD have a relatively slow rate of decline and timing of listing for transplantation is difficult. While many will have type II respiratory failure with all that that implies for prognosis, there are a large group of patients whose life is at a standstill in terms of severe functional restriction but who nevertheless have areasonable prognosis as judged from their spirometry and blood gas estimations. If these patients do not have other significant contraindications it is reasonable to list them for transplantation on the basis that they will gain improvement in quality of life if not in survival. It should be clearly explained to these patients that they are exchanging the risks and uncertainties of the post-transplantation course for this improvement in quality of life alone.

The availability of LVRS has, if anything, tightened the indications for lung transplantation. Those patients who are in particular not hypercapnic or pulmonary hypertensive may well be offered volume reduction surgery, whereas those who have obvious contraindications to LVRS (see below) are more likely to be acceptable candidates for lung transplantation. Having decided the patient is eligible on physiological or prognostic grounds, a number of important contraindications must be excluded (Table 8.5). The common reasons for refusing or delaying transplantation acceptance include renal impairment (because of intolerance to cyclosporin or tacrolimus in the post-operative phase), osteoporosis – common following long-term steroids and lack of physical exercise – and coronary artery disease. Most patients over the age of 55, and younger if they have an elevated cholesterol or a positive family history, should undergo coronary angiography. In practice the yield of significant disease is relatively small. Osteoporosis is common and we would regard a 'Z score' of more than 2 standard deviations from the predicted normal for the age to be a contraindication. These patients all become more osteopenic in the post-operative phase as a result of the catabolic state and the increased steroid dosage.

Selection of procedure

Most patients with COPD will be listed for single lung transplantation (SLTx). This procedure gives a very satisfactory functional improvement, is a straightforward procedure and achieves the economy of donor organs.

Evidence of bilateral sepsis, with chronic sputum production and perhaps CT appearances of established bronchiectasis are a contraindication to SLTx and such patients should be considered for the bilateral procedure. They compete very directly with the large number of cystic fibrosis patients requiring bilateral lung transplantation.

Table 8.5 Contraindications for lung transplantation in patients with COPD

ABSOLUTE
Severe non-pulmonary organ dysfunction
Renal deficiency. Glomerular filtration rate < 40 ml/h
Coagulopathy or borderline hypertension
Left ventricular dysfunction (any cause)
Severe coronary artery disease (consider heart and lung transplantation)
Cancer (other than skin) within the last 5 years
Active extrapulmonary infection
HIV
Hepatitis B (surface antigen positive)
Hepatitis C
Severe psychiatric illness: continued drug dependence
Severe malnutrition, body mass index <16
Severe obesity, body mass index >30

RELATIVE
Osteoporosis
Hypertension
Diabetes
Significant pre-operative steroid dose (particularly with side-effects)
Intubation and ventilation
Previous thoracic surgery including pleurodesis
Chronic pulmonary infection (may require bilateral lung transplantation)
Age >60 years

However, many of those patients are of relatively small stature and the more normal sized, together with the greatly enlarged chest cavity, mean that lungs from relatively tall donors can be used for this group whereas they not be suitable for the CF patients.

The presence of coronary disease or left ventricular dysfunction would indicate the need for heart–lung transplantation but in practice these patients so often have other co-morbidities that they are no longer accepted for lung transplantation.

Surgical procedure

SLTx is performed through a lateral thoracotomy with anastomoses of bronchus, pulmonary vein and pulmonary artery. Bronchial healing is ensured by a short donor bronchus and end-to-end apposition of the bronchial mucosa. Telescoped anastomoses or wrapping with extraneous tissues such as vascularised omentum is no longer considered necessary (Wilson *et al.* 1996).

The major problem in the post-operative period is relative over-expansion of the contralateral recipient lung. The transplant lung always has impaired compliance and there is inevitably a tendency for air trapping in the severely emphysematous residual lung. The transplant lung has no lymphatics, a tendency to alveolar collapse and almost inevitably has a degree of endothelial injury with neutrophil trapping and the substrate for acute respiratory distress syndrome. The key practical difficulty is the inability to apply positive end-expiratory pressure (PEEP) to the transplant lung without suffering air trapping in the residual lung. The resultant scenario is a progressive overinflation of the residual lung and collapse of the transplant lung. It can be obviated by periods of double-lumen ventilation, often leaving the native lung unventilated and open to air (Smiley *et al.* 1991). This strategy re-expands the transplant lung and eliminates $\dot{V}/\dot{Q}$ (i.e. ventilation–perfusion) matching. Nitric oxide is of proven benefit if there is donor lung dysfunction (Date *et al.* 1996).

Results of lung transplantation for COPD

Peri-operative mortality for all lung transplant recipients is between 7 and 10 per cent with a one-year survival rate of 75 per cent and a five-year survival rate of 45 per cent in published registries. There is some evidence that patients with emphysema do a little better in the early phases than other diagnostic groups. The surgical procedure is more straightforward and one-year survival rates as high as 90 per cent are being recorded from single institutions. The most reliable data, however, are those from validated registries. In the United Kingdom all pulmonary transplantations are recorded by the Intrathoracic Audit Database run under the auspices of the Royal College of Surgeons. One-year survival rate for UK patients undergoing SLTx is 75 per cent.

Costs and benefits of lung transplantation for emphysema

As has already been suggested, the natural history of patients with COPD is relatively more benign than for other groups of patients undergoing lung transplantation. This is clearly demonstrated in the curves published by Hosenpud *et al.* (1998), from UNOS data in the United States (Figure 8.4). In this paper, there was no demonstrable survival advantage for lung transplantation for emphysema compared with survival rate on the waiting list. The principal determinant of who receives the transplant is time on the waiting list and thus the emphysema patients are particularly suited to survive up to the time of their transplantation. The ISHLT data, largely reflecting United States experience, shows that 62 per cent of all pulmonary transplantations were performed for emphysema. The figure in the UK is much lower, at 23 per cent. This figure demonstrates the pragmatic approach of many UK centres in transplanting the sickest patients and ignoring time on the waiting list as a significant factor.

Bilateral lung versus single lung

On the ISHLT registry, 79 per cent of patients with emphysema received a unilateral transplantation (Hosenpud *et al.* 2000). Some centres have reported a better short-term survival for the bilateral lung transplantation (Bavaria *et al.* 1997) and there are a number of reported better long-term survivals (Sundaresan *et al.* 1996). In the

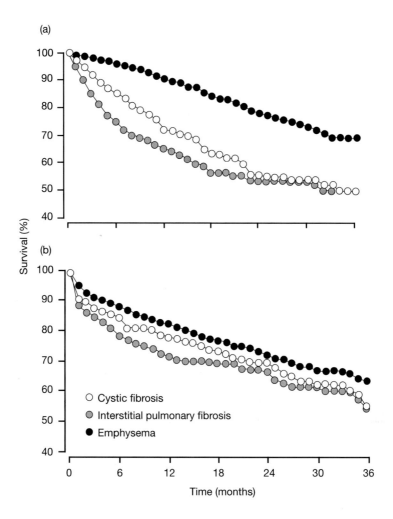

Figure 8.4 (a) Emphysema patients have a lower attrition rate on the waiting list. (b) Their survival post-transplantation is no different than pre-transplantation. From Hosenpud *et al.* (1998) with permission © The Lancet Ltd 1998

registry data there is a small but significant separation of survival curves to the advantage of the bilateral group after three years. On the other hand, it must be remembered that most patients selected for bilateral lung transplantation are younger and were selected because of their perceived need for their greater exercise capacity. It is difficult to reconcile the relatively 'expensive' use of paired lung transplantation for patients anticipating quality of life rather than survival benefits. This is a particularly difficult argument when it is remembered that most of the other groups competing for paired lung transplantations have a survival advantage from transplantation.

Conclusions

Both of these surgical approaches for patients with emphysema have significant limitations. Transplantation can only ever be applied to a small number of patients, particularly in competition with other other diagnostic groups. Long-term function remains limited by obliterative bronchiolitis.

Candidates for volume reduction surgery are now better defined, but the inevitable decline of function with time, although to be expected, is a disappointment. The relative costs and benefits, in terms of both morbidity and finance, have yet to be ascertained.

References

Bavaria JE, Kotloff R, Palevsky H *et al.* (1997). Bilateral versus single lung transplantation for chronic obstructive pulmonary disease. *Journal of Thoracic and Cardiovascular Surgery* **113**, 520–528

Brantigan O, Kress M, Mueller E (1959). A surgical approach to pulmonary emphysema. *American Review of Respiratory Disease* **39**, 19–202

Brenner M, McKenna Jr RJ, Chen JC *et al.* (1999). Survival following bilateral staple lung volume reduction surgery for emphysema. *Chest* **115**, 390–396

Cassina PC, Teschler H, Konietzko N *et al.* (1998). Two-year results after lung volume reduction surgery in α-1 antitrypsin deficiency versus smoker's emphysema. *European Respiratory Journal* **12**, 1028–1032

Cooper JD, Pearson FO, Patterson GA *et al.* (1987). Technique of successful lung transplantation in humans. *Journal of Thoracic and Cardiovascular Surgery* **93**, 173–178

Cooper JD, Trulock EP, Triantafillou AN *et al.* (1995). Bilateral pneumonectomy (volume reduction) for chronic obstructive pulmonary disease. *Journal of Thoracic and Cardiovascular Surgery* **109**, 106–116

Cooper JD, Patterson GA, Sundaresan RS *et al.* (1996). Results of 150 consecutive bilateral lung volume reduction procedures in patients with severe emphysema. *Journal of Thoracic and Cardiovascular Surgery* **112**, 1319–1330

Cranshaw J & Evans TW (2001). Lung volume reduction surgery: a quality operation? *Lancet* **357**, 650–651

Criner GJ, Cordova GC, Furukawa S *et al.* (1999). Prospective randomized trial comparing bilateral lung volume reduction surgery to pulmonary rehabilitation in severe chronic obstructive pulmonary disease. *American Journal of Respiratory & Critical Care Medicine* **160**, 2018–2027

Date H, Triantafillou AN, Trulock EP *et al.* (1996). Inhaled nitric oxides reduces human allograft dysfunction. *Journal of Thoracic and Cardiovascular Surgery* **111**, 913–919

Deslauriers J (1996). History of surgery for emphysema. *Seminars in Thoracic and Cardiovascular Surgery* **8**, 43–51

Flaherty KR & Fernando JM (2000). Lung volume reduction surgery for emphysema. *Clinics in Chest Medicine* **21**, 819–848

Gaensler EA, Cugell DW, Knudson RJ *et al.* (1983). Surgical management of emphysema. *Clinics in Chest Medicine* **4**, 443–463

Geddes D, Davies M, Koyama H *et al.* (2000). Effect of lung volume reduction surgery in patients with severe emphysema. *New England Journal of Medicine* **343**, 239–245

Gelb AF, McKenna RJ, Brenner M *et al.* (1999). Lung function after bilateral lower lobe lung volume reduction surgery for α-1 antitrypsin emphysema. *European Respiratory Journal* **14**, 928–933

Hamacher J, Bloch KE, Satmmberger U *et al.* (1999).Two years outcome of lung volume reduction in different morphological emphysema types. *Annals of Thoracic Surgery* **68**, 1792–1798

Hazelrigg SR, Boley TM, Magee MJ *et al.* (1998). Comparison of staged thoracoscopy and median sternotomy for lung volume reduction surgery. *Annals of Thoracic Surgery* **66**, 1134–1139

Hosenpud JD, Bennett LE, Keck BM *et al.* (1998). Effect of diagnosis on survival benefit of lung transplantation for end-stage lung disease. *Lancet* **351**, 24–27

Hosenpud JD, Bennett LE, Keck BM *et al.* (1999). The registry of the International Society for Heart and Lung Transplantation: Sixteenth official report. *Journal of Heart and Lung Transplantation* **18**, 611–626

Hosenpud JD, Bennett LE, Keck BM, Boucek MM, Novick R (2000). The registry of the International Society for Heart and Lung Transplantation: Seventeenth official report. *Journal of Heart and Lung Transplantation* **19**, 909–931

Keenan RJ, Landrenau RJ, Sciurba FC *et al.* (1996). Unilateral thoracoscopic surgical approach for diffuse emphysema. *Journal of Thoracic and Cardiovascular Surgery* **111**, 308–316

Kotloff RM, Tino G, Bavaria JE *et al.* (1996). Bilateral lung volume reduction surgery for advanced emphysema. A comparison of median sternotomy and thorascopic approaches. *Chest* **110**, 1399–1408

McKenna RJ Jr, Brenner M, Fischel RJ *et al.* (1996a). Should lung volume reduction for emphysema be unilateral or bilateral. *Journal of Thoracic and Cardiovascular Surgery* **112**, 1331–1338

McKenna RJ, Brenner M, Gelb AF *et al.* (1996b). A randomized, prospective trial of stapled lung reduction versus laser bullectomy for diffuse emphysema. *Journal of Thoracic and Cardiovascular Surgery* **111**, 317–322

Mal H, Andreassian B, Fabrice P *et al.* (1989). Unilateral lung transplantation in end-stage pulmonary emphysema. *American Review of Respiratory Diseases* **140**, 797–802

Meyers BF, Yusen RD, Lefrak SS *et al.* (1998). Outcome of Medicare patients with emphysema selected for, but denied, a lung volume reduction operation. *Annals of Thoracic Surgery* **66**, 331–336

Miller JI, Lee RB, Mansour KA (1996). Lung volume reduction surgery: Lessons learned. *Annals of Thoracic Surgery* **61**, 1464–1469

Naunheim KS, Keller CA, Krucylak PE *et al.* (1996). Unilateral video-assisted thoracic surgical lung reduction. *Annals of Thoracic Surgery* **61**, 1092–1098

Ojo TC, Martinez FJ, Paine R III *et al.* (1997). Lung volume reduction surgery after management of pulmonary nodules in patients with severe COPD. *Chest* **112**, 1494–1500

Pompeo E, Marino M, Nofroni I *et al.* (2000). Reduction pneumoplasty versus respiratory rehabilitation in severe emphysema: A randomized study. *Annals of Thoracic Surgery* **70**, 948–954

Reitz BA, Wallwork JL, Hunt SA *et al.* (1982). Heart-lung transplantation: successful therapy for patients with pulmonary vascular disease. *New England Journal of Medicine* **306**, 559–64

Smiley RM, Navedo AT, Kirby T *et al.* (1991). Postoperative independent lung ventilation in a single-lung transplant recipient. *Anesthesiology* **74**, 1144–1148

Stevens PM *et al.* (1970). Regional ventilation and perfusion in patients after lung transplantation. *New England Journal of Medicine* **232**, 245–8

Sundaresan RS, Shiraishi Y, Trulock EP *et al.* (1996). Single or bilateral lung transplantation for emphysema? *Journal of Thoracic and Cardiovascular Surgery* **112**, 1485–95

Wakabayashi A (1995). Thoracoscopic laser pneumoplasty in the treatment of diffuse bullous emphysema. *Annals of Thoracic Surgery* **60**, 936–942

Wilson IC, Hasan A, Healy M, Villaquiran J *et al.* (1996). Healing of the bronchus in pulmonary transplantation. *European Journal of Cardiothoracic Surgery* **10**, 521–527

Wisser W, Tschernko E, Senbaklavaci O *et al.* (1997). Functional improvement after volume reduction: Sternotomy versus videoendoscopic approach. *Annals of Thoracic Surgery* **63**, 822–828

Young J, Fry-Smith A, Hyde C (1999). Lung volume reduction surgery (LVRS) for chronic obstructive pulmonary disease (COPD) with underlying severe emphysema. *Thorax* **54**, 779–789

PART 4

Evidence and opinion for managing disability and progressing rehabilitation

Chapter 9

A strategy for the management of disability and the reduction of handicap in COPD

Michael DL Morgan and Michael C Steiner

Introduction

Chronic obstructive pulmonary disease (COPD) is characterised by progressive airflow obstruction that eventually becomes symptomatic, producing cough, wheeze and breathlessness. Early changes may have little impact on function or quality of life but eventually the progression of the disease leads to substantial personal disability and handicap. The progression of illness and growing healthcare burden may also have major consequences for the family and the wider community. The airflow obstruction that initiates the illness cannot usually be reversed and therapeutic strategies are limited to reduction of symptoms, improvement in functional capacity and limitation of the social impact. This chapter will examine the role of rehabilitation and environmental adaptation in achieving these aims.

The development of disability and handicap in COPD

Progression of dyspnoea in COPD is associated with a chain of events that leads to disability that is not wholly the result of the underlying airway obstruction. Patients enter a spiral of decline that involves avoidance of activity, skeletal muscle de-conditioning, loss of confidence and isolation (Figure 9.1). This implies that improvement can be obtained by reversal or attenuation of these factors alone. COPD is a good model for the application of the World Health Organization definitions of impairment, disability and handicap (World Health Organization 1980). In the context of COPD, impairment is represented by the pathophysiology such as reduction in forced expiratory volume in 1 second (FEV_1), fat-free mass or $Vo_{2peak.}$ Disability represents the consequent loss of functional capacity and handicap is the social impact. These definitions are currently under review but still provide a useful model for therapeutic ambition. In general, the impairments are relatively easy to measure but difficult to change. By contrast, features of disability and handicap may be more difficult to assess but may offer more opportunity for improvement. Pulmonary rehabilitation reduces disability by improving individual symptoms and functional performance. A reduction in handicap requires changes to lifestyle and adaptation of the physical and social environment.

Dyspnoea

Adaptation

Avoidance

Inactivity

De-conditioning

Isolation   Disability

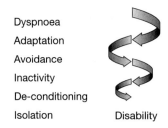

Figure 9.1 The development of disability in COPD

Assessment of disability and handicap

As COPD develops, FEV_1 declines and becomes a less useful outcome assessment. Measures of health status, functional performance, domestic activity and health economics are more relevant to the aims of rehabilitation. These measures have now been adapted or developed for clinical use.

Reduced exercise performance is the consequence of dyspnoea that leads to disability. Physical performance in COPD can be assessed by clinical examination, formal questionnaire, field exercise tests or laboratory examination. Clinician assessment of exercise performance is unreliable and physicians are inaccurate judges of performance (Oren *et al.* 1987). Simple questionnaires such as the MRC dyspnoea scale are a blunt but reliable reflection of performance (Bestall *et al.* 1999). Objective laboratory exercise testing is the most thorough method of assessment but may not be readily available. Field exercise tests are a suitable substitute for laboratory and can be standardised. Examples of walking tests that have been used in rehabilitation are the six-minute walk test and the incremental and endurance shuttle walk tests (Singh *et al.* 1992; Revill *et al.* 1999).

Assessment of handicap requires more subtlety than measuring impairment or physical performance. Many of the components of handicap can be improved by reversing impairment or reducing disability while others require society to adapt to the patients' needs. Some reflection of handicap can be obtained from health status measures, particularly the disease-specific questionnaires. Examples that have demonstrated sensitivity to rehabilitation are the Chronic Respiratory Questionnaire (CRQ), the Breathing Problems Questionnaire (BPQ), and St George's Respiratory Questionnaire (SGRQ) (Hyland *et al.* 1998; Guyatt *et al.* 1999; Griffiths *et al.* 2000). Although these questionnaires broadly reflect handicap they do contain elements of impairment and disability in their structure. There is only one questionnaire, the PAIS-SR, that claims to cover only aspects of handicap and has been used for patients with COPD. Interestingly it does appear to uncover aspects of social deprivation that have not been previously identified by health professionals (Stubbing *et al.* 1998).

Apart from the quality of life questionnaires there are also a number of functional status questionnaires that report on activities of daily living (ADL). Some of these have been designed for people with lung disease (PFSS and PFSDQ) while others have been adapted from ADL scores derived from people with other disabilities. It is also possible to use physical activity monitors to count daily activity, although the true value of this is uncertain (Steele *et al.* 2000).

Managing disability

Improving the wider disability in COPD involves a sequence that begins with smoking cessation and medical reversal of impairment wherever possible. Later, improvement of individual disability can be achieved by a process of rehabilitation including physical training and psychological and social support (Figure 9.2). Addressing the residual handicap may then require social adaptation.

The evidence for benefit of pulmonary rehabilitation is now growing and has been published in a number of reviews and guidelines (ACCP/AACVPR Pulmonary Rehabilitation Guidelines Panel 1997; American Thoracic Society 1999). The summary of this evidence suggests that a multi-professional, individually tailored programme should improve physical function, dyspnoea and health status, and have health economic advantages (Figure 9.3). This recommendation is now based on the highest quality of evidence (Petrie *et al.* 1995). Details of the necessary processes of rehabilitation are gradually becoming understood. There are important issues surrounding the selection of candidates, the content and duration of the activity and the site of the programme.

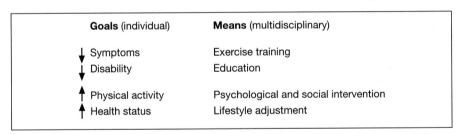

Goals (individual)	**Means** (multidisciplinary)
↓ Symptoms	Exercise training
↓ Disability	Education
↑ Physical activity	Psychological and social intervention
↑ Health status	Lifestyle adjustment

Figure 9.2 The aims of pulmonary rehabilitation

Evidence exists that a multi-professional, individually tailored, programme of rehabilitation including prescribed endurance exercise training should:

• Improve functional capacity (walking distance)	Grade A
• Improve health status	Grade A
• Reduce dyspnoea	Grade A
• Reduce hospital stay and GP call-outs	Grade A

Figure 9.3 The benefits of pulmonary rehabilitation

Selection for rehabilitation

In general the benefits of rehabilitation appear to apply to all those with disabling dyspnoea due to chronic lung disease. The timing of rehabilitation may not be that easy to judge but should be determined by the level of symptoms and not by a pre-set threshold of impairment. There is little evidence for discrimination on the basis of age, impairment, starting disability or even smoking status. In fact, patients with severe disability may have proportionately more to gain from the process. In practice the real barriers to effective rehabilitation are the pragmatic issues of geography, availability of transport and the presence of co-morbid conditions such as arthritis or dementia that make physical training difficult.

Programme content and duration

Physical exercise

To obtain benefit the programmes must contain some form of lower limb physical training of adequate intensity. In practice, this usually involves periods of individually prescribed, supervised, brisk walking or static cycle exercise. Exclusion of lower limb exercise from the programme negates the overall benefit. The benefits of physical training include improved exercise performance and health status. However, the two benefits do not necessarily correlate. The mechanism for improvement in exercise performance following rehabilitation is complex and not simply related to physiological training, although this may occur. Other factors such as improvement in confidence, technique or pacing may also play a part and increased self-efficacy may be the link between improved physical performance and health status. Genuine physiological training may be possible in many patients with COPD, although demonstration of this effect may be more difficult than in healthy subjects. Improvements in anaerobic threshold may not be demonstrable in people with a ventilatory limit to exercise (Casaburi *et al.* 1991; Maltais *et al.* 1997). However, there is now muscle biopsy evidence of physiological training adaptation with increases in oxidative enzymes following rehabilitation. Obviously the effectiveness of training will increase with the training intensity but this will be offset by the risk of intolerance or injury. As a rule, exercise prescription should be individually set at the highest sustainable intensity and gradually increased with tolerance. Some benefits will be obtained even in those who can only achieve a modest training load.

Apart from lower limb endurance training, other possible modalities include strength, upper limb exercise and respiratory muscle training. These modes of training do not result alone in the global improvements of health status and exercise performance. However, improved peripheral muscle strength may well improve the wider disability as a component of other functions (Simpson *et al.* 1992; Clark *et al.* 2000). There is also a rationale for upper limb training to improve the ability to perform domestic activities but this form of training is task specific and does not confer wider benefits. Training of the respiratory muscles may seem a profitable approach but also does not yet appear to confer wider benefit beyond the task. There is a possibility that the combination of higher intensity respiratory muscle training and general aerobic exercise training may have an additive effect (Berry *et al.* 1996). All rehabilitation programmes contain lower limb training and many will add strength or upper limb exercises while the inclusion of respiratory muscle training is not currently to be recommended.

Other components

Disease education is a central component of rehabilitation even though it has not been shown to have any independent beneficial effect (Toshima *et al.* 1990). Nevertheless it is assumed that disease education must have a role in facilitating the rehabilitation process and is also likely to help the understanding of carers and relatives. Suggested components of an educational series would include disease education, dietary advice, technical issues (oxygen, nebulisers, etc.), relaxation, sexuality and benefits advice.

The value of formal psychological, social or behavioural intervention is not clear. It could be imagined that such techniques could affect anxiety, depression and coping skills, or improve the affective component of dyspnoea. There is currently no evidence of major benefit for psychotropic medication or group therapy in this area. There may, however, be some role for behavioural techniques in improving self-efficacy.

Individual physiotherapy tuition may be helpful for sputum clearance where appropriate but formal efforts to change patterns of breathing have no lasting effect (Gosselink *et al.* 1995). General advice about nutrition and healthy eating is also welcome. Some people with COPD are obese and will benefit from weight reduction while others are malnourished. There is a relationship between reduction in fat free mass and mortality in COPD and it is tempting to consider this as a potentially reversible factor (Schols *et al.* 1998; Landbo *et al.* 1999). However, recent examination of the evidence suggests that nutritional supplementation alone has no effect (Ferreira *et al.* 2000). For the present the available evidence is insufficient and further investigation of the role of nutritional supplements in association with different anabolic stimuli is required.

Site, duration and provision of rehabilitation programmes

The site of rehabilitation does not seem to be critical. Successful programmes have been described as hospital inpatients, hospital outpatients, community centres and in patients' homes. Minor differences in effectiveness between the sites have been identified but the major choice in venue will be determined by the cost. Inpatient programmes are expensive and the best value appears to be the hospital outpatient version.

The optimum duration of suitable rehabilitation programmes also seems to be variable. Long-lasting benefits of exercise performance and health status have been recorded following six weeks of outpatient rehabilitation (Griffiths *et al.* 2000). These benefits can be retained for 12–18 months without further maintenance (Singh *et al.* 1998; Guell *et al.* 2000). The minimum period of rehabilitation necessary to achieve results is not known but it is likely that the positive outcomes of physical reconditioning and health status improvement may require different timescales. The role of maintenance or repeat therapy is also uncertain. Whether prolonged rehabilitation has any benefit is uncertain. Programmes exceeding 12 weeks do not seem to confer additional advantage (Criner *et al.* 1999). Comparison of maintenance programmes with limited duration rehabilitation has not been made but when maintenance is performed it does not need to be frequent (Vogiatzis *et al.* 1999).

The provision of pulmonary rehabilitation in the United Kingdom is poor. There is no culture of provision and little encouragement from purchasers to provide a service in spite of the good scientific evidence. Hopefully, this situation will alter with the acknowledgement of the benefits and the pressure from consumer groups to resource services. The realisation of the real costs of COPD care may also help highlight the issue.

Addressing handicap in COPD

Once optimal medical management has been achieved and the patient has undergone pulmonary rehabilitation there may still be residual wider disability or handicap that cannot be reduced by attention to the individual. In this case attention can be paid to adapting the environment around the patient to reduce the impact of the disease (Figure 9.4). This might range from the provision of simple equipment to enhance performance to the adaptation of the home. On a wider scale, handicap may also be reduced by the greater provision of social services and the political campaigning for more resources.

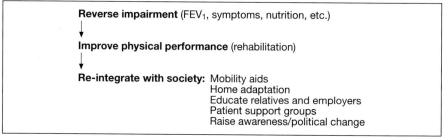

Figure 9.4 COPD: managing disability and reducing handicap

Individual assessment of pure handicap may be difficult and not always particularly useful. The only pure estimate of handicap that is available is the PAIS-SR since other health status measures also cover the other domains of wider disability. In one trial the PAIS-SR did uncover higher levels of handicap than were perceived by health professionals. Physical aids to mobility can have a significant impact. These include ambulatory oxygen and wheeled walking aids which can improve walking distance significantly (Honeyman *et al.* 1996; Revill *et al.* 2000). Other home adaptations such as stair lifts and occupational therapy aids or re-housing may also have a role following appropriate assessment.

One thing that appears to disadvantage patients with COPD is the lack of perception of true disability. The significant problems of disability and handicap in people with COPD are often not clear to the observer in the way that might be obvious in other physical disabilities. This perception is often voiced by patients and there is also some evidence that COPD patients with equivalent levels of disability to those with physical deformities do not receive the same degree of social service support (Yohannes *et al.* 1998).

Redressing the balance of healthcare provision for people with COPD may require political action. Patient support groups such as Breathe Easy (British Lung Foundation) are beginning to develop campaigning skills to influence commissioners and purchasers of health care. This might operate at a local level through the public meetings of the health authorities and primary care trusts. Alternatively patients can seek to influence national policy through politicians and government. Either way there are strong arguments for redressing the balance for people with COPD whose disability and handicap has not been recognised or addressed. An accurate assessment of the true costs of COPD to the wider community may help facilitate this process.

References

ACCP/AACVPR Pulmonary Rehabilitation Guidelines Panel (1997). Pulmonary rehabilitation: joint ACCP/AACVPR evidence-based guidelines. American College of Chest Physicians. American Association of Cardiovascular and Pulmonary Rehabilitation [see comments]. *Chest* **112**, 1363–1396

American Thoracic Society (1999). Pulmonary rehabilitation – 1999. *American Journal of Respiratory & Critical Care Medicine* **159**, 1666–1682

Berry MJ, Adair NE, Sevensky KS, Quinby A, Lever HM (1996). Inspiratory muscle training and whole-body reconditioning in chronic obstructive pulmonary disease. *American Journal of Respiratory & Critical Care Medicine* **153**, 1812–1816

Bestall JC, Paul EA, Garrod R, Garnham R, Jones PW, Wedzicha JA (1999). Usefulness of the Medical Research Council (MRC) dyspnoea scale as a measure of disability in patients with chronic obstructive pulmonary disease. *Thorax* **54**, 581–586

Casaburi R, Patessio A, Ioli F, Zanaboni S, Donner CF, Wasserman K (1991). Reductions in exercise lactic acidosis and ventilation as a result of exercise training in patients with obstructive lung disease [see comments]. *American Review of Respiratory Disease* **143**, 9–18

Clark CJ, Cochrane LM, Mackay E, Paton B (2000). Skeletal muscle strength and endurance in patients with mild COPD and the effects of weight training. *European Respiratory Journal* **15**, 92–97

Criner GJ, Cordova FC, Furukawa S *et al.*(1999). Prospective randomized trial comparing bilateral lung volume reduction surgery to pulmonary rehabilitation in severe chronic obstructive pulmonary disease. *American Journal of Respiratory & Critical Care Medicine* **160**, 2018–2027

Ferreira IM, Brooks D, Lacasse Y, Goldstein RS (2000). Nutritional support for individuals with COPD: a meta-analysis. *Chest* **117**, 672–678

Gosselink RA, Wagenaar RC, Rijswijk H, Sargeant AJ, Decramer ML (1995). Diaphragmatic breathing reduces efficiency of breathing in patients with chronic obstructive pulmonary disease. *American Journal of Respiratory & Critical Care Medicine* **151**, 1136–1142

Griffiths TL, Burr ML, Campbell IA *et al.* (2000). Results at 1 year of outpatient multidisciplinary pulmonary rehabilitation: a randomised controlled trial. *Lancet* **355**, 362–368

Guell R, Casan P, Belda J *et al.* (2000). Long-term effects of outpatient rehabilitation of COPD: A randomized trial. *Chest* **117**, 976–983

Guyatt GH, King DR, Feeny DH, Stubbing D, Goldstein RS (1999). Generic and specific measurement of health-related quality of life in a clinical trial of respiratory rehabilitation. *Journal of Clinical Epidemiology* **52**, 187–192

Honeyman P, Barr P, Stubbing DG (1996). Effect of a walking aid on disability, oxygenation, and breathlessness in patients with chronic airflow limitation. *Journal of Cardiopulmonary Rehabilitation* **16**, 63–67

Hyland ME, Singh SJ, Sodergren SC, Morgan MD (1998). Development of a shortened version of the Breathing Problems Questionnaire suitable for use in a pulmonary rehabilitation clinic: a purpose-specific, disease-specific questionnaire. *Quality of Life Research* **7**, 227–233

Landbo C, Prescott E, Lange P, Vestbo J, Almdal TP (1999). Prognostic value of nutritional status in chronic obstructive pulmonary disease. *American Journal of Respiratory & Critical Care Medicine* **160**, 1856–1861

Maltais F, LeBlanc P, Jobin J *et al.*(1997). Intensity of training and physiologic adaptation in patients with chronic obstructive pulmonary disease. *American Journal of Respiratory & Critical Care Medicine* **155**, 555–561

Oren A, Sue DY, Hansen JE, Torrance DJ, Wasserman K (1987). The role of exercise testing in impairment evaluation. *American Review of Respiratory Disease* **135**, 230–235

Petrie J, Barnwell B, Grimshaw J, on behalf of the Scottish Intercollegiate Guidelines Network (1995). *Clinical Guidelines: Criteria for appraisal for national use.* Edinburgh: Royal College of Physicians

Revill SM, Morgan MD, Singh SJ, Williams J, Hardman AE (1999). The endurance shuttle walk: a new field test for the assessment of endurance capacity in chronic obstructive pulmonary disease. *Thorax* **54**, 213–222

Revill SM, Singh SJ, Morgan MD (2000). Randomized controlled trial of ambulatory oxygen and an ambulatory ventilator on endurance exercise in COPD. *Respiratory Medicine* **94**, 778–783

Schols AM, Slangen J, Volovics L, Wouters EF (1998). Weight loss is a reversible factor in the prognosis of chronic obstructive pulmonary disease. *American Journal of Respiratory & Critical Care Medicine* **157**, 1791–1797

Simpson K, Killian K, McCartney N, Stubbing DG, Jones NL (1992). Randomised controlled trial of weightlifting exercise in patients with chronic airflow limitation. *Thorax* **47**, 70–75

Singh SJ, Morgan MD, Scott S, Walters D, Hardman AE (1992). Development of a shuttle walking test of disability in patients with chronic airways obstruction. *Thorax* **47**, 1019–1024

Singh SJ, Smith DL, Hyland ME, Morgan MD (1998). A short outpatient pulmonary rehabilitation programme: immediate and longer-term effects on exercise performance and quality of life. *Respiratory Medicine* **92**, 1146–1154

Steele BG, Holt L, Belza B, Ferris S, Lakshminaryan S, Buchner DM (2000). Quantitating physical activity in COPD using a triaxial accelerometer. *Chest* **117**, 1359–1367

Stubbing DG, Haalboom P, Barr P (1998). Comparison of the Psychosocial Adjustment to Illness Scale-Self Report and clinical judgment in patients with chronic lung disease. *Journal of Cardiopulmonary Rehabilitation* **18**, 32–36

Toshima MT, Kaplan RM, Ries AL (1990). Experimental evaluation of rehabilitation in chronic obstructive pulmonary disease: short-term effects on exercise endurance and health status. *Health Psychology* **9**, 237–252

Vogiatzis I, Williamson AF, Miles J, Taylor IK (1999). Physiological response to moderate exercise workloads in a pulmonary rehabilitation program in patients with varying degrees of airflow obstruction. *Chest* **116**, 1200–1207

World Health Organization (1980). *International Classification of Impairments, Disabilities and Handicaps*. Geneva: World Health Organization

Yohannes AM, Roomi J, Connolly MJ (1998). Elderly people at home disabled by chronic obstructive pulmonary disease. *Age & Ageing* **27**, 523–525

PART 5

Effectiveness and efficiency in the delivery and improvement of clinical services

Chapter 10

A critical appraisal of published clinical practice guidelines for the investigation and management of COPD and the relevance of the guidelines of the Global initiative for Obstructive Lung Disease (GOLD) to routine clinical practice in the UK

Nicola Stevenson and Peter Calverley

Introduction

In the last decade there has been a renewed appreciation of the importance of chronic obstructive pulmonary disease (COPD) as a cause of morbidity and mortality in both the developed and the developing world (Office of Population Censuses and Surveys 1993; Anderson *et al.* 1994; Murray & Lopez 1997a, 1997b). At the same time, it was recognised that the production of management guidelines for diseases such as bronchial asthma increased the quality and consistency of care. As a result, a large number of national and international guidelines for the diagnosis and management of COPD have been published. It would be impossible to conduct a detailed comparison of these in the space available here. Instead this chapter will focus on the principal similarities and some differences between these existing management approaches and the newly developed Global initiative for Obstructive Lung Disease (GOLD) guidelines which will soon be available for widespread application. Although this may not be as comprehensive as desirable, it is unlikely to omit any important differences as the majority of national guidelines have been greatly influenced by the European Respiratory Society and American Thoracic Society publications. The British Thoracic Society guidelines have also had wide impact beyond the UK and these will be contrasted with the others.

Existing guideline documents

The first published guidelines for the management of chronic pulmonary disease were those of the Canadian Thoracic Society in 1992 (Canadian Thoracic Society Workshop Group 1992). They were relatively brief and consensus-based, being formulated by an expert panel and submitted to the Society for approval. They summarised currently accepted views about existing treatments but did not particularly suggest a scheme for management. The approach adopted by the

European Respiratory Society and published three years later (The European Respiratory Society Task Force 1995) was more comprehensive, giving more detail about the disease and a clear definition that emphasised physiological impairment as an important diagnostic criterion (see below). These guidelines were developed by a series of expert panels and included recommendations about staging and disease management. The flow charts produced to illustrate this have proven difficult to adapt in differing medical environments and although intended as the centrepiece of the management section they have not been widely implemented. The American Thoracic Society developed standards of care recommendations for COPD (American Thoracic Society 1987) which were really an extension of an area statement of appropriate standards of care updated in 1995. The resulting document was extremely comprehensive, particularly for hospitalised COPD patients. The British Thoracic Society published its guidelines in 1997 (COPD Guidelines Group for the Standards of Care Committee of the BTS 1997) and to date this is the only one that has involved general physicians, nurse specialists, emergency medicine physicians and patient support groups in its production. Like the other documents it was developed by a core writing group who held meetings with this wider constituency and from the resulting feedback and dialogue with the editors of *Thorax* a generally more useable approach was developed. Specific targets and thresholds were included which were intended to promote particular actions by relevant medical groups, e.g., criteria for admission to hospital or referral to the outpatient clinic. This may explain why this approach has been adopted beyond the national audience for which it was originally produced.

All of these guideline documents with the exception of those of the Canadian Thoracic Society, which has recently been revised, are still in their first edition. Since the guidelines were developed in the early 1990s, there has been increasing sophistication in their application and many regulatory authorities no longer rely on selective citation of the evidence in favour of a particular treatment approach but wish to see how strong that evidence is. The information on which these documents were based was largely that available in the early 1990s and in the interval several significant changes have occurred that impact on COPD management. For this reason, it appeared timely to seek a more systematic approach to COPD guidelines and one which could be readily updated. This process led directly to GOLD.

Global initiative for Obstructive Lung Disease (GOLD)

The GOLD process arose as a result of the successful Global Initiative in Asthma (GINA) which had been launched through a collaboration between the World Health Organization and the National Heart Lung and Blood Institute in the USA. Although basically developed by pulmonary experts from around the world and without the extensive consultation with family medicine and nurses groups, which characterised the BTS approach, the GOLD guidelines are intended to have widespread applicability. This has meant that some specific issues such as the relative roles of physicians, nurse specialists and others have not been included in the current document. However, it is anticipated that regionally based physician documents will be developed which are more didactic than the present general review and which are applicable to specific healthcare systems elsewhere in the world. Finally, a patient booklet will be produced which will again be specific to particular cultures and reflect the availability of healthcare while retaining evidence-based recommendations.

Several different systems of grading evidence have been developed and the one used in GOLD is listed in Figure 10.1. This falls short of a full-scale systematic

Evidence category	Sources of evidence	Definition
A	Randomised controlled trials (RCTs) Rich body of data	Evidence is from endpoints of well-designed RCTs that provide a consistent pattern of findings in the population for which the recommendation is made. Category A requires substantial numbers of studies involving substantial numbers of participants
B	Randomised controlled trials Limited body of data	Evidence is from endpoints of intervention studies that include only a limited number of RCTs, post-hoc or subgroup analysis of RCTs, or meta-analysis of RCTs. In general, category B pertains when few randomised trials exist, they are small in size, the results are somewhat inconsistent, or they were undertaken in a population that differs from the target population of the recommendation
C	Non-randomised trials Observational studies	Evidence is from outcomes of uncontrolled or non-randomised trials or from observational studies
D	Panel consensus judgement	This category is used only in cases where the provision of some guidance was deemed valuable but the clinical literature addressing the subject was deemed insufficient to justify placement in one of the other categories. The Panel Consensus is based on clinical experience or knowledge that does not meet the above-listed criteria

Figure 10.1 Description of levels of evidence

review of evidence in each area which was beyond the resources of this project. Moreover, not all aspects of COPD management can be graded in this way and there are large areas, particularly those relating to diagnosis, where there is no clinical trial evidence to support the use of one approach rather than another. In many cases, it is unlikely that specific clinical trials to assess the utility of procedures will be conducted and so level D evidence is likely to remain the best available.

All of the guidelines contain some general background about the pathophysiology of COPD but more detail about the epidemiology, health impacts and economic burden of COPD is provided in the GOLD document. Although intended to be generally applicable, it is clear that these data are currently dominated by trans-Atlantic information and there is an urgent need, highlighted in the research recommendations, to acquire systematic data in developing countries. Before considering therapy, there are two general areas where differences are worth highlighting.

BTS	Chronic obstructive pulmonary disease is a chronic, slowly progressive disorder characterised by airflow obstruction (reduced FEV_1 and FEV_1/VC ratio) that does not change markedly over several months. Most of the lung function impairment is fixed, although some reversibility can be produced by bronchodilator (or other) therapy
GOLD	COPD is a disease characterised by progressive airflow limitation that is not fully reversible. It is associated with an abnormal inflammatory response of the lungs to noxious particles or gases

Figure 10.2 BTS and GOLD definitions of COPD

Defining COPD

All of the major national and international guidelines now define COPD in terms of clinical symptoms and the presence of airflow limitation. This has been defined by an FEV_1/VC (or FVC) ratio, which is reduced below 70 per cent. The definition of COPD used in GOLD does not specify this exactly as this is within the body of the document, but it does emphasise two further features. Firstly, that COPD is usually a progressive disorder and secondly that it arises as a result of persisting inflammation and that this is due to inhalation of noxious particles or gases. This clearly separates COPD from bronchial asthma, at least in terms of aetiology and, by emphasising the inflammatory component, raises the prospect that future therapeutic intervention might be possible. Figure 10.2 illustrates the BTS and GOLD definitions.

Approaches to diagnosis

All the guidelines are agreed that spirometry is the best and most reproducible way of assessing both the severity of COPD and confirming the diagnosis. There is widespread agreement that measuring post-bronchodilator FEV_1 is the most robust endpoint, while the role of bronchodilator reversibility testing remains controversial. The GOLD guidelines emphasise that decisions about therapy with bronchodilator drugs should not be made on the basis of bronchodilator testing, a point first noted in the BTS guidelines. The criteria for a positive response to this test may be relevant to the prescription of inhaled corticosteroids but there is no agreement between the major guidelines as to what such a response should be. GOLD recommends the ATS criterion (American Thoracic Society 1995) of a 12 per cent improvement in FEV_1 after a bronchodilator, which exceeds 200 ml. The ERS believes a response constitutes bronchodilator improvement which is >10 per cent of the predicted normal FEV_1 for that individual. The BTS suggests that the increase from baseline should be 15 per cent and at least 200 ml. Each of these definitions has significant weaknesses and there are data that reproducibility from day to day is not good (Tweedale *et al.* 1987). Primary care physicians have found that undertaking bronchodilator reversibility is of limited value as well as being time consuming. The best reasons for doing these tests are to determine the post-bronchodilator FEV_1 which does have prognostic value and identification of those patients with a substantial improvement, i.e., more than two standard deviations beyond the between-day reproducibility of FEV_1. This group of patients can show substantial improvements in FEV_1 during therapy with inhaled corticosteroids (Nisar *et al.* 1992) but probably account for <10 per cent of the total number of COPD patients attending hospital.

A further difference between guidelines is in the staging system. Limitations of FEV_1 as a guide to symptoms have been emphasised from data gathered using health status questionnaires (Jones *et al.* 1992; Hajiro *et al.* 1999) and as a result the GOLD guidelines have adopted deliberately broad bands in terms of staging severity by FEV_1. There is no doubt that the lower the individual's post-bronchodilator FEV_1 then the more severe is the accompanying lung disease. However, this does not predict either the degree of symptom limitation or the efficacy of therapy. The GOLD staging system is more concerned with public health issues and includes an 'at risk' group of people where the FEV_1 is >80 per cent but there are symptoms of regular cough and sputum production and exposure to a known risk factor such as cigarette smoking. These at-risk people can be identified for the specific early intervention. Mild disease is present if the FEV_1 is between 70 and 80 per cent predicted with an obstructive ratio and moderate severity encompasses the 30–70 per cent predicted FEV_1 group. Within this range a number of treatments are considered but the need for them is decided on the severity of the patients' symptoms. Once the FEV_1 is below 30 per cent predicted and/or there is evidence of respiratory failure with an arterial P_{O_2} breathing air below 8 kPa then other therapies are to be considered as both the mortality and the risk of hospitalisation rise sharply. This approach differs from other staging systems based on FEV_1, where considerations of prognosis, rather than symptomology, have dominated the classification. However, all of these staging systems are artificial and are really designed as an aid to introducing therapy. It is the lack of success in convincing practical clinicians of the need to anchor all their treatments to arbitrary specified values of FEV_1 that led to the different approach adopted in GOLD.

Chronic disease management

Both the BTS and the GOLD guidelines outline the goals of therapy (Figure 10.3). These remain the benchmarks against which the effects of any treatment should be judged. No single treatment achieves all of these and in COPD, unlike asthma, reduction in the age-related rate of deterioration, rather than complete abolition of symptoms, is the best that we can currently aspire to. The following topics are addressed in all the guidelines.

GOLD guidelines: objectives of chronic management

- Relief of symptoms
- Improvement of lung function
- Decrease of exacerbations
- Decrease of hospitalisations
- Improvement of quality of life
- Inhibition of lung function decline
- Increase of life expectancy

Figure 10.3 GOLD guidelines: objectives of chronic management

Smoking cessation

Although universally recommended, only the GOLD guidelines make clear recommendations about the use of nicotine replacement therapy and its role in an integrated smoking cessation strategy. They comment favourably on the possibility of using Bupropion as a further agent to smoking cessation (Jorenby *et al.* 1999). The benefits of smoking cessation are supported by ample grade A evidence (Connett *et al.* 1993; United States Department of Health and Human Services *et al.* 1990) but, as GOLD points out, there are other known environmental factors that contribute to COPD and withdrawal from these may involve a change of either occupation or legislation.

Bronchodilator therapy

All the guidelines recommend bronchodilators on a regular basis, but reviewing the recent studies the GOLD guidelines are more supportive of a specific role for long-acting inhaled β agonists (Jones & Bosh 1997; Mahler *et al.* 1999). There are preliminary data that long-acting inhaled anticholinergics when they are licensed will also be of considerable value. The inhaled route is always preferred because of its favourable side-effects profile and short acting β agonists are thought to have a more rapid onset than anticholinergics and for this reason are the preferred rescue therapy. The essence of the GOLD approach is to encourage persistent use of bronchodilator drugs either four times daily, if short-acting drugs are given, or twice daily if long-acting β agonists are employed. To date there are no clear differences between salmeterol and eformoterol in this respect (Maeson et al. 1999).

Inhaled corticosteroids

The role of inhaled corticosteroids has been unclear as pointed out in both the ERS and ATS statements. The BTS approach has been to suggest that these drugs be reserved for patients who show positive response to oral corticosteroid trials. This perhaps identifies around 10 per cent of COPD patients and the GOLD guidelines suggest that it may be preferable to use a longer course of inhaled corticosteroids as the risks of persistent and inadvertent oral therapy are thereby avoided (Callahan et al. 1991; Decramer et al. 1994; Pauwels et al. 1999). The GOLD guidelines also have the benefit of the more recent large studies of inhaled corticosteroids in a range of COPD severity. There is no evidence that these drugs modify the rate of decline in lung function with time (Pauwels et al. 1999; Vestbo et al. 1999), but in patients with more severe disease they reduce the number of exacerbations and reduce the impact of the disease on the patient's health over time (Burge et al. 2000). Thus, GOLD recommends (grade B evidence) that these drugs be used on patients with more severe disease who have a history of frequent exacerbations. There is increasing evidence that oral corticosteroids are harmful and should not be used for maintenance treatment.

Other treatments

There is still controversy over the role of mucolytic and anti-oxidant drugs in COPD with evidence from meta-analysis that these drugs can reduce the number of episodes of chronic bronchitis (Poole & Black 2000). Whether these data are comparable to those seen with inhaled corticosteroids remains unclear and, as these drugs are not licensed in all countries, GOLD recommendations in this area will be neutral.

Anti-tussives and leukotriene modifiers are not recommended as there is no significant evidence yet of benefit with these agents in COPD.

In contrast, there is a wealth of evidence at grade A level supporting the role for pulmonary rehabilitation. Unlike the BTS guidelines, where this was restricted to patients with more severe disease, it is now recognised that patients can benefit from pulmonary rehabilitation at any stage in their illness when they have developed symptoms of exercise limitation and breathlessness. The exercise component remains the most important aspect (Rees 1990) and there is evidence that patients undergoing rehabilitation have fewer exacerbations and less hospitalisation (Rees 1990; Griffiths et al. 2000). The role of domiciliary oxygen is predominantly in patients with persistent hypoxaemia where it can prolong life, while the data for oxygen during exercise are more mixed and the groups who benefit most are not well defined (Nocturnal Oxygen Therapy Trial Group 1980; Medical Research Council Working Party 1981). While vaccination against influenza can be strongly recommended from large studies, nasal ventilation remains an experimental therapy.

Surgical treatment of bullae has strong grade C evidence in its support but the picture regarding lung volume reduction surgery is less clear-cut. The large North American Emphysema Treatment trial is ongoing and its results regarding cost benefit will be awaited with interest. There are more recent data, however, which confirm the efficacy of this form of surgery in relatively mixed COPD populations. Lung transplantation is an effective form of palliation, which does not prolong life.

Managing acute exacerbations

Both GOLD and the British Thoracic Society provide clear guidance relevant to family physicians about when hospitalisation should be considered. All of the guidelines agree that there is a definite role of oxygen in patients who are hospitalised. Nebulised bronchodilators are also recommended (Moayyedi et al. 1995; Friedman 1997). Antibiotics may benefit those cases where there is cough and green sputum production (Anthonisen et al. 1987). GOLD has benefited from the availability of two recent randomised control studies confirming an important place for oral corticosteroids in the treatment of acute exacerbations of COPD, but suggesting that there is no advantage in prolonged therapy (Davies et al. 1999; Niewoehner et al. 1999). Another new treatment, which has now got a much better evidence base and is addressed in GOLD, is non-invasive positive pressure ventilation. This provides an acceptable alternative to conventional positive pressure ventilation at least in patients with arterial pH >7.25 (Plant et al. 2000). GOLD provides some guidance about whom this treatment should help and what the indications are. Like the BTS, the GOLD guidelines have tried to specify those criteria that should be met before a patient is discharged home, and to emphasise that there should be some kind of discharge treatment plan. These data represent panel consensus, but can provide an important way of improving patient care.

The future

One of the major concerns of the GOLD guidelines Panel has been to ensure not only that the evidence is summarised but that it leads to a scheme of treatment that can be implemented. The implementation phase of GOLD is only just beginning but if it follows the pattern of the GINA guidelines it will have significant effects, particularly in countries that were previously not considered in need of such co-ordinated treatment. For countries like the UK where there are already established recommendations, the GOLD data provide a way of updating current practice. At present it is not clear when the next revision of the BTS Guidelines will take place, but it is probable that this will not occur within the next 12–18 months. The recommendations in GOLD are therefore more up to date and current than any likely to be made on a national basis in the next two years and should be considered when planning local service development. One of the features of the GOLD approach is that it is adaptable to national countries' perceptions and if clinical consensus suggests a more stratified approach to treatment there is no real conflict with the aims of GOLD. What is important is that COPD should be recognised as an important cause of ill health where valuable therapies are available. Practical ways should be sought to implement these varied treatment approaches in an individualised and co-ordinated way, which will benefit patients. As new data emerge all these recommendations need to be reconsidered and the balance of evidence in certain areas is likely to change either for or against particular practices. One final feature of GOLD, which is potentially valuable, is that it will be available on the internet and it will be updated in a regular way as new information becomes available. This is likely to be the future for all forms of guideline documents which should greatly simplify the process of ensuring that up-to-date information is readily available to practising clinicians.

References

American Thoracic Society (1987). Standards for the diagnosis and care of patients with chronic obstructive pulmonary disease (COPD) and asthma. *American Review of Respiratory Disease* **136**, 225–244

American Thoracic Society (1995). Standards for the diagnosis and care of patients with chronic obstructive pulmonary disease. *American Journal of Respiratory & Critical Care Medicine* **152**, 577–620

Anderson HR, Esmail A, Hollowell J *et al.* (1994). *Epidemiologically Based Needs Assessment: Lower Respiratory Disease.* London: Department of Health

Anthonisen NR, Manfreda J, Wairen CP, Hershfield ES, Harding GK, Nelson NA (1987). Antibiotic therapy in exacerbations of chronic obstructive pulmonary disease. *Annals of Internal Medicine* **106**, 196–204

Burge PS, Calverley PMA, Jones PW, Spencer S, Anderson JA, Maslen TK (2000). Randomised double blind placebo controlled study of fluticasone propionate in patients with moderate to severe COPD: The ISOLDE Trial. *British Medical Journal* **320**, 1297–1303

Callahan CM, Dittus RS, Katz BP (1991). Oral corticosteroid therapy for patients with stable chronic obstructive pulmonary disease. A meta-analysis. *Annals of Internal Medicine* **114**, 216–223

Canadian Thoracic Society Workshop Group (1992). Guidelines for the assessment and management of chronic obstructive pulmonary disease. *Canadian Medical Association Journal* **147**, 420–428

Connett JE, Kusek JW, Bailey WC, O'Hara P, Wu M (1993). Design of the Lung Health Study: a randomised clinical trial of early intervention for chronic obstructive pulmonary disease. *Controlled Clinical Trials* **14**, s3–19

COPD Guidelines Group for the Standards of Care Committee of the BTS (1997). BTS guidelines for the management of chronic obstructive pulmonary disease. *Thorax* **52**, 51–52

Davies L, Angus RM, Calverley PMA (1999). Oral corticosteroids in patients admitted to hospital with exacerbations of COPD: a prospective randomised controlled trial. *Lancet* **354**, 456–460

Decramer M, Lacquet LM, Fagard R, Rogiers P (1994). Corticosteroids contribute to muscle weakness in chronic airflow obstruction. *American Journal of Respiratory & Critical Care Medicine* **150**, 11–16

European Respiratory Society Task Force (1995). Optimal assessment and management of chronic obstructive pulmonary disease. *European Respiratory Journal* **8**, 1398–420

Friedman M (1997). Combined bronchodilator therapy in the management of chronic obstructive pulmonary disease. *Respirology* **2**, s19–23

Griffiths TL, Burr ML, Campbell IA *et al.* (2000). Results at 1 year of out-patient multidisciplinary pulmonary rehabilitation. *Lancet* **355**, 362–368

Hajiro T, Nishimura K, Tsukino M, Ikeda A, Oga T, Izumi T (1999). A comparison of the level of dyspnea vs disease severity in indicating the health-related quality of life of patients with chronic obstructive pulmonary disease. *Chest* **116**, 1632–1637

Jones PW & Bosh TK (1997). Quality of life changes in COPD patients treated with salmeterol. *American Journal of Respiratory & Critical Care Medicine* **155**, 1283–1289

Jones PW, Quirk FH, Baveystock CM, Littlejohns P (1992). A self-complete measure of health status for chronic airflow limitation. The St. George's Respiratory Questionnaire. *American Review of Respiratory Disease* **145**, 1321–1327

Jorenby DE, Leischow SJ, Nides MA *et al.* (1999). A controlled trial of sustained-release bupropion, a nicotine patch, or both for smoking cessation. *New England Journal of Medicine* **340**, 685–691

Maesen BL, Westermann CJ, Duurkens VA, van de Bosch JM (1999). Effects of fomoterol in apparently poorly reversible chronic obstructive pulmonary disease. *European Respiratory Journal* **13**, 1103–1108

Mahler DA, Donohue JF, Barbee RA *et al.* (1999). Efficacy of salmeterol xinafoate in the treatment of COPD. *Chest* **115**, 957–965

Medical Research Council Working Party (1981). Long term domiciliary oxygen therapy in chronic hypoxic cor pulmonale complicating chronic bronchitis and emphysema. Report of the Medical Research Council Working Party. *Lancet* **i**, 681–686

Moayyedi P, Congleton J, Page RL, Pearson SB, Muers MF (1995). Comparison of nebulised salbutamol and ipratropium bromide with salbutamol alone in the treatment of chronic obstructive pulmonary disease. *Thorax* **50**, 834–837

Murray CJ & Lopez AD (1997a). Alternative projections of mortality and disability by cause 1990-2020: Global Burden of Disease Study. *Lancet* **349**, 1498–1504

Murray CJ & Lopez AD (1997b). Mortality by cause for eight regions of the world: Global Burden of Disease Study. *Lancet* **349**, 1269–1276

Niewoehner DE, Erbland ML, Deupree RH *et al.* (1999). Effect of systemic glucocorticoids on exacerbations of COPD. *New England Journal of Medicine* **340**, 1941–1947

Nisar M, Earis JE, Pearson MG, Calverley PMA (1992). Acute bronchodilator trials in chronic obstructive pulmonary disease. *American Review of Respiratory Disease* **146**, 555–559

Nocturnal Oxygen Therapy Trial Group (1980). Continuous or nocturnal oxygen therapy in hypoxaemic chronic obstructive lung disease: a clinical trial. *Annals of Internal Medicine* **93**, 391–398

Office of Population Censuses and Surveys (1993). *Mortality Statistics, Causes: England and Wales 1992; Series DH2 No 19.* London: HMSO

Pauwels RA, Lofdahl C-G, Laitinen LA *et al.* (1999). Long term treatment with inhaled budesonide in persons with mild chronic obstructive pulmonary disease who continue smoking. *New England Journal of Medicine* **340**, 1948–1953

Plant PK, Owen JL, Elliott MW (2000). Early use of non-invasive ventilation for acute exacerbations of chronic obstructive pulmonary disease on general respiratory wards: a multicentre randomised controlled trial. *Lancet* **355**, 1931–1935

Poole PJ & Black PN (2000). Mucolytic agents for chronic bronchitis or chronic obstructive pulmonary disease. *Cochrane Database of Systemic Reviews* **2**, CD001287

Rees AL (1990). Position paper of the American Association of Cardiovascular and Pulmonary Rehabilitation: Scientific basis of pulmonary rehabilitation. *Journal of Cardio Pulmonary Rehabilitation* **10**, 418–441

Tweedale PM, Alexander F, McHardy GJR (1987). Short term variability in FEV1 and bronchodilator responsiveness in patients with obstructive ventilatory defects. *Thorax* **42**, 87–90

United States Department of Health and Human Services (1990). *The Health Benefits of Smoking Cessation: A Report of the Surgeon General.* Rockville, MD: Public Health Service, Centers for Disease Control. Publication No. CDC 90-8416

Vestbo J, Sorensen T, Lange P, Brix A, Torre P, Viskum IC (1999). Long-term effect of inhaled budesonide in mild and moderate COPD: a randomised controlled trial. *Lancet* **353**, 1819–1823

Organising the provision of effective palliative care services for patients with advanced chronic obstructive pulmonary disease

Carol L Davis

Introduction

Thirteen per cent of adult disability in the United Kingdom in 1986 was caused by chronic respiratory diseases, mostly chronic obstructive airway disease (COPD) (Royal College of Physicians 1986). It has been calculated that, in an average health district, COPD accounts for 1,000 admissions and 25,000 primary care consultations per annum (Strachan 1995). COPD also accounts for 6.4 per cent of all male deaths and 3.9 per cent of all female deaths (British Thoracic Society 1997). Per annum, about 28,000 patients die of COPD in England and Wales, a number that is remarkably similar to that of deaths from lung cancer (Office of Population and National Statistics 1999). The three-year mortality rate of patients with hypoxic COPD in the Medical Research Council randomised controlled trial of long-term oxygen therapy was 45 per cent in the treatment arm and 67 per cent in the control arm (Medical Research Council Oxygen Working Party 1981). Although this mortality rate is high, it is lower than for lung cancer which, sadly, is still 95 per cent at five years.

Palliative care has been defined in various ways. The most widely adopted definition was devised by the World Health Organization in 1990: 'palliative care is the active, total care of patients whose disease is not responsive to curative treatment. Control of pain, of other symptoms, and of psychological, social and spiritual problems is paramount. The goal of palliative care is the best quality of life for patients and their families.' More recently, the National Council for Hospice and Specialist Palliative Care Services (1995) has suggested definitions of the terms 'palliative care', 'palliative care approach' and 'specialist palliative care services' (Figure 11.1). The philosophy that underpins palliative care revolves around the concept of living with disease rather than dying of disease and terminal care is but one part, albeit an important one, of palliative care. Palliative care services have traditionally been provided for patients with cancer but some services have accepted referrals of patients with non-malignant disease for many years. In the last ten years, increasing numbers of hospice and palliative care services have been resourced to extend their services to either selected patients with non-malignant disease, most

---

Palliative care
Palliative care is the active total care of patients and their families by a multi-professional team when the patient's disease is no longer responsive to curative treatment.

The palliative care approach
The palliative care approach aims to promote both physical and psychosocial well being. It is a vital and integral part of all clinical practice, whatever the illness or its stage, informed by a knowledge and practice of palliative care principles.

Specialist palliative care services
Specialist palliative care services are those services with palliative care as their core speciality. Specialist palliative care services are needed by a significant minority of people whose deaths are anticipated, and may be provided:

- directly through the specialist services;
- indirectly through advice to a patient's present professional advisers/carers.

Figure 11.1 Definitions

often motor neuron disease and HIV disease, or appropriate patients with any potentially life-threatening non-malignant disease.

Despite this, the national survey of hospice and hospital palliative care services in 1997–1998 demonstrated that approximately 95 per cent of hospice inpatient and patients referred to hospital palliative care services have cancer. Given that 75 per cent of people in the UK die of non-malignant disease, it has been argued that the provision of palliative care services for people with diagnoses other than cancer is both inequitable and inadequate (National Council for Hospice and Specialist Palliative Care Services 1998).

Palliative care and patients with non-malignant disease

There is evidence that conventional care may not be meeting the palliative care needs of patients with non-malignant disease adequately (Hockley *et al.* 1988; Addington-Hall & McCarthy 1995a, 1995b). The Regional Study of the Care of the Dying was a large retrospective survey of the views of bereaved relatives and friends of the last year of life (Addington-Hall & McCarthy 1995a, 1995b). The response rate was 69 per cent and two-thirds of respondents were the bereaved relatives of patients with cancer. Seventeen per cent of the 3,696 interviews conducted with non-cancer patients indicated that the patients had suffered symptoms equal in severity or number to the one-third of cancer patients who received specialist palliative care and had the most severe and numerous symptoms. None of the former had received specialist palliative care.

A large American study, the SUPPORT study, has also demonstrated palliative care needs across a range of diseases including several non-malignant ones (Lynn *et al.* 1997). The researchers found that 40 per cent of dying patients suffer pain at least half of the time across all disease categories.

Palliative care needs of patients with advanced COPD

Two recent studies have addressed the palliative care needs of patients with advanced COPD.

In Doncaster, a palliative care needs assessment was conducted in patients with advanced COPD who were aged over 55 years and had been admitted to hospital with an acute exacerbation for seven days or more in the last six months (Skilbeck *et al.* 1998). The methods included in-depth interviewing, quality of life assessment and assessment of resource use. The chosen quality-of-life tools were the European Organization for the Research and Treatment of Cancer (EORTC) core questionnaire and lung cancer module which are not validated in patients with COPD – a limitation of the study. Over a 21-month period (1995–1997) the response rate was 63 of 151 (42 per cent). A poor quality of life was demonstrated with a high prevalence of

Table 11.1 Most frequent physical symptoms (EORTC quality-of-life data) in patients with COPD

Symptom	n	%
Extreme breathlessness	60	95
Pain	43	68
Fatigue	43	68
Difficulty sleeping	34	55
Thirst	34	54

- Symptom management
- Support in daily activities
- Emotional support
- Social support
- Information

Figure 11.2 Main palliative care needs of patients with advanced COPD

symptoms (Table 11.1), a high degree of social isolation and emotional distress, low physical functioning and significant disability. The patients' needs identified from the interviews are summarised in Figure 11.2. These are unlikely to be substantially different from the palliative care needs of patients with cancer.

These findings are in line with a more recent study: an open, comparative study of palliative care and quality of life in 100 patients, half with severe COPD and half with unresectable non-small cell lung cancer (NSCLC), reported by Gore *et al.* (2000). This revealed that the patients with COPD had more significantly impaired quality of life in terms of emotional social and physical functioning, more unrecognised psychological problems and more unmet information needs than patients with NSCLC. The authors concluded that patients with end-stage COPD have palliative care needs that remain unaddressed, and that many have needs that parallel those of patients with lung cancer. The accompanying editorial in *Thorax* discusses issues about quality of life in patients with COPD and those with lung cancer and voices some concern about the nature of the patient populations and other methodological issues in the Gore paper (Hill & Muers 2000). None the less, the comparative study is a very useful addition to the literature on this subject.

With the exception of pulmonary rehabilitation programmes, much of current service provision for people with COPD is geared towards the crisis management of acute exacerbations in either primary or secondary care. 'Hospital at home' initiatives are already proving successful at preventing acute hospital admissions, but may not address chronic problems such as breathlessness, anxiety and panic, or provide ongoing emotional and social support. It seems likely that unmet palliative care needs exist, which, in some patients, will include specialist palliative care needs.

Potential models of specialist palliative care service delivery

In the Policy Framework for Commissioning Cancer Services, Calman stated that: 'It is the responsibility of every healthcare professional to provide palliative care, and to call in specialist colleagues if the need arises, as an integral component of good clinical practice, whatever the illness or its stage' (National Health Service Executive 1994). The evidence reviewed in this paper, along with common sense and principles of equity, support the extrapolation of this statement to patients with COPD. The challenge to those who currently care for patients with COPD and to specialist palliative care services (SPCS) is to devise a workable system that avoids duplication of effort, ensures efficient and appropriate communication between all involved, and optimises the quality of life for patients with advanced COPD without overwhelming the patient and their family with well-intentioned professionals.

Whilst much palliative care for patients with COPD should continue to be delivered by primary care, respiratory and general medical teams through a palliative care approach, a framework is needed whereby specialist palliative care advice and support can be available when appropriate, whether the patient is at home, in a residential or nursing home, a community hospital or acute hospital. The fact that the increasing numbers of clinical nurse specialists and nurse consultants in respiratory care will make a significant contribution to the palliative care of patients with COPD must be borne in mind when predicting the specialist palliative care needs of patients with COPD. Some potential models of service delivery are shown in Figure 11.3.

- Hands-off advice

- One-off consultative visits

- Short-term involvement

- Longer-term involvement

Figure 11.3 Specialist palliative care service delivery: potential models

One solution might be to provide a telephone advisory service for healthcare professionals caring for patients with advanced COPD. This would have relatively small resource implications for SPCS but would have the distinct disadvantage that, without patient contact, specialist palliative care professionals would have little opportunity to build up their knowledge and skills about this patient group. An alternative strategy might be one-off consultative visits ideally with a primary care or respiratory team healthcare professional with knowledge of both that patient and the disease. This could be impractical for those working in primary or secondary care and, in practice, a telephone discussion between the relevant professionals rather than a joint consultation is likely to be the norm. Some patients with specific specialist palliative care needs may need short-term involvement of a palliative care team alongside other healthcare and social care professionals. Shared care with the general practitioner and primary care team or hospital team is essential. A few patients might require longer-term involvement of SPCS. Whichever model is feasible and appropriate at a local level, flexibility of service provision is required. The natural history of COPD is progressive disability with intermittent acute exacerbations. The author does not think that it is appropriate for palliative care professionals to care for patients with COPD during infective exacerbations and, in any case, palliative care services would be swamped by demand. None the less it is likely that some patients may require intermittent episodes of specialist palliative care intervention. Specialist palliative care services comprise support in the community, day care, inpatient care in a specialist palliative care unit, hospital palliative care team input and bereavement services. Admission and discharge criteria for each of these aspects will need to be devised jointly by SPCS and others involved in the care of these patients and their families.

Challenges for specialist palliative care

Professionally, we are moulded by our knowledge, skills and attitudes. For specialist palliative care professionals these attributes will have developed predominantly through their training and experience with patients with cancer, and may not be transferable to patients with COPD. On the other hand, many palliative care principles apply to any patient with progressive disease, especially those who are dying. There is no doubt, however, that there will be learning needs and a learning curve as specialist palliative care extends its services to these patients. In particular, the author feels that it is likely that specialist palliative care could learn much from pulmonary rehabilitation and that such knowledge will be referable to a significant proportion of patients with advanced malignant disease.

If specialist palliative care services are to be provided to selected patients with COPD it is essential that groundrules, and perhaps protocols, are established in conjunction with general practitioners and the respiratory team. For example, palliative care physicians are well used to prescribing relatively high doses of dexamethasone for a range of specified clinical problems in patients with cancer, but a more modest dose of prednisolone may be far more appropriate, when necessary, in a patient with COPD.

It is always difficult, and sometimes impossible, to estimate prognosis in patients with cancer. In patients with COPD, prognosis may be even more unpredictable particularly if a palliative care professional without expert knowledge of the COPD disease process or longitudinal contact with that patient tries to prognosticate. This has clinical and resource implications because an informed guess about prognosis is frequently an important part of clinical decision-making.

Knowledge, skills and attitudes appropriate to this patient population will develop in palliative care professionals so long as they are able to work alongside other healthcare professionals with expertise in the care of patients with COPD. Even so, a steady flow of patients rather than, say, one or two referrals per annum, may be required to build their experience.

Patients are admitted to specialist palliative care units for symptom control (including psychological problems), rehabilitation, respite or terminal care. Most units do not have the capacity to admit patients with cancer for respite on a regular basis, although such a service may allow patients to remain at home by relieving stress and lay carer burden. It is likely that there will be increasing demand for respite admissions for patients with COPD. This could have significant resource implications including an effect on bed occupancy and waiting lists but, in any case, may not be appropriate. A specialist palliative care unit in which the majority of patients have advanced cancer, the staff are mainly experienced in caring for patients with cancer and approximately 50 per cent of admissions result in death not discharge may not be an appropriate care setting for patients with COPD. It will be important to decide which patients with respite needs also have specialist palliative care needs.

For those without specialist needs, hospice admission is likely to be the wrong course of action. The author believes that specialist palliative care could not and should not prop up the inadequate and over-pressed social care provision in the United Kingdom. Admissions for other reasons may be appropriate after discussion with all involved.

Lastly, it is important to remember that many specialist palliative care units, and professionals, especially nurses, are funded to care for patients with cancer. In particular, those funded by cancer charities, including Macmillan Cancer Relief and Marie Curie Cancer Care, have a responsibility to those charities to care, in the main, for patients with cancer.

Personal reflection

Recently, I was asked to see a 75-year-old, deaf man with long-standing COPD and cor pulmonale. He had been in hospital for several weeks having been admitted with an infective exacerbation of COPD and marked renal impairment. Treatment had comprised intravenous rehydration, antibiotics, diuretics and nasal intermittent positive pressure ventilation, and he was much improved. I was, in my capacity as consultant on the Hospital Palliative Care Team, asked to see him in the high care respiratory ward to advise on his breathlessness. After the consultation, I wrote in his medical notes: 'We explored issues about his breathing, episodes of severe breathlessness and associated anxiety/panic, living with an incurable disease and his coping strategies. In particular we talked about non-drug strategies for acute breathlessness and panic.' I said that I would review him in a few days if he was still an inpatient.

When I went to review him, I saw that the SHO had written '?WRONG PATIENT' underneath my entry in the notes. Why was this? Had I misinterpreted what the patient had told me? Had the patient told me things that either he had not had the chance to tell the respiratory team or had chosen not to? Was the SHO so preoccupied with serial renal function and blood gas results that he was unaware of the man's main concerns? Had I got more time to spend with him than my colleagues? Did my palliative care experience and the fact that I was not involved in his day-to-day care allow me to focus on different issues than others? Was the SHO more in tune with the main problems than me? It is difficult to know. When I saw the patient again, he initiated the conversation and told me that some of the things I had suggested had helped, that he appreciated seeing 'a proper doctor without an entourage' and that he was worried about how his wife would cope when he died. We discussed all these feelings in some detail.

He was discharged soon after and I have not seen him again or heard how he is getting on. I like to think that my consultations with him may have had some lasting benefit. But that's something else that I don't know and probably never will.

Conclusions

The title of this chapter presupposes that patients with advanced COPD have palliative care and specialist palliative care needs. The author believes this to be true but, just as all patients with advanced cancer do not have specialist palliative care needs, nor do all patients with advanced COPD. Specialist palliative care does not have a monopoly on caring, on good listening skills or even on best possible symptom control nor should it. In selected patients, however, involvement of specialist palliative care services alongside pre-existing services in primary care and acute hospitals may bring a different focus on a patient's problems and thus may generate new ideas as to ways of addressing those problems.

Despite increased interest in the palliative care of patients with non-malignant disease, and of those with COPD in particular, relatively little has been written, or perhaps even discussed, about the best way to provide effective palliative care services for these patients. Most patients' palliative care needs will continue to be addressed by the primary care and respiratory teams. For those with specialist palliative care needs it seems likely that no single model of service delivery will address the needs of this population and their lay and professional carers. Instead, a variety of models may need to be employed in different localities and in different patients. Moreover, since the appropriateness of any service intervention varies not only between patients but also over time in any one patient, flexibility and an openness of all professionals involved in that patient's care to review the patient's needs and the best ways to address them regularly, will be required. These service developments will provide ample opportunity for research and audit. Indeed, at least initially, appropriate evaluation from several different perspectives should be mandatory.

Education of palliative care specialists about patients with COPD and COPD specialists about palliative care will also be essential. It has been said that a true specialist is one who recognises their own limits of ignorance. To date, the author has been involved in the care of patients with COPD only in the acute hospital setting, even though she sees patients with cancer in the community and hospice as well as the acute hospital. The hospital setting seems to me to be a relatively easy place to learn more about the nature of COPD and its effect on patients because there are respiratory colleagues to talk to, learn from and discuss ideas with. There is no doubt that specialist palliative care also has a lot to learn from primary care about this group of patients.

Team-working across professions, specialties and healthcare settings can be challenging but within this challenge lies the key to the provision of effective palliative care services for patients with COPD. Within a team, professionals need to acknowledge both their individual boundaries and areas of overlap. By so doing, all involved should be able to maintain appropriate, professional roles in maintaining, and where possible improving, the quality of life and death of patients with advanced COPD without becoming 'Jacks of all trades and masters of none', and without crowding out the patient and their family.

References

Addington-Hall J & McCarthy M (1995a). Dying from cancer: results of a national population based investigation. *Palliative Medicine* **9**, 295–230

Addington-Hall J & McCarthy M (1995b). Regional study of care for the dying: methods and sample characteristics. *Palliative Medicine* **9**, 27–35

British Thoracic Society (1997). BTS guidelines for the management of chronic obstructive pulmonary disease. *Thorax* **52**, S5

Gore JM, Brophy CJ, Greenstone MA (2000). How well do we care for patients with end stage chronic obstructive pulmonary diseases (COPD)? A comparison of palliative are and quality of life in COPD and lung cancer. *Thorax* **55**, 1000–1006

Hill KM & Muers MF (2000). Palliative care for patients with non-malignant end stage respiratory disease. *Thorax* **55**, 979–981

Hockley JM, Dunlop R, Davies RJ (1988). Survey of distressing symptoms in dying patients and their families in hospital and the response to a symptom control team. *British Medical Journal* **296**, 1715–1717

Lynn J, Teno JM, Phillips RS *et al.* (1997). Perceptions by family members of the dying experience of older seriously ill patients. *Annals of Internal Medicine* **126**, 97–106

Medical Research Council Oxygen Working Party (1981). Long-term domiciliary oxygen therapy in chronic hypoxic cor pulmonale complicating chronic bronchitis and emphysema. *Lancet* **i**, 681–685

National Council for Hospice and Specialist Palliative Care Services (1995). *Specialist Palliative Care: A Statement of Definitions. Occasional Paper 8*

National Council for Hospice and Specialist Palliative Care Services (1998). *Reaching Out: Specialist Palliative Care for Adults with Non-Malignant Diseases. Occasional Paper 14*

National Health Service Executive (1994). *A Policy Framework for Commissioning Cancer Services*. London: Department of Health

Office of Population and National Statistics (1999). *Annual Report*. London: HMSO

Royal College of Physicians (1986). Physical disability in 1986 and beyond. *Journal of the Royal College of Physicians* **3**, 160–194

Skilbeck J, Mott L, Page H, Smith D, Hjelmeland-Ahmedzai S, Clark D (1998). Palliative care in chronic obstructive airways disease: a needs assessment. *Palliative Medicine* **12**, 245–254

Strachan DP (1995). Epidemiology: a British perspective. In: Calverley P, Pride N (eds) *Chronic Obstructive Pulmonary Disease*. London: Chapman & Hall, pp 47–67

World Health Organization (1990). *Cancer Pain Relief and Palliative Care (Technical Report Series 804)*. Geneva: World Health Organization

Common medical errors and their classification in the investigation and management of COPD

Mike G Pearson

Introduction

Chronic obstructive pulmonary disease (COPD) is a huge burden to the health service. Some 600,000 people in the UK have COPD and up to 10 per cent of all acute medical admissions are due to COPD (Pearson *et al.* 1994). Until the advent of guidelines from the British Thoracic Society (1997) there was no consensus as to how these patients should be managed and thus it was not possible to define or describe errors in management since no one knew what an error was. The Guidelines set out a framework within which to manage COPD: they are not prescriptive and do not set out a protocol. Thus the title of this chapter might better be termed 'Comon medical problems …' rather than 'Common medical errors ...' since that is what is being described. The word 'error' implies that someone has been at fault and that is too strong a word given present knowledge.

There are many problems that could be described but this chapter will concentrate on just five major areas:

- not confirming the diagnosis;
- misinterpretation of symptoms and their causation;
- not relating treatment to severity;
- too many given nebulisers;
- too few offered non-invasive ventilation (NIV) rescue.

Not confirming the diagnosis

The diagnosis of COPD was defined in clinico-pathological terms in the COPD guidelines (Figure 12.1). The British Guidelines were the first to include specific reference to altered spirometry as part of the definition, although all the major national and international versions agree that it is essential to have an objective confirmation of the diagnosis. In primary care, spirometry is only available in some practices and there was an awareness among those producing their guidelines that this might be a problem. Accordingly a survey was commissioned to ascertain primary care knowledge of COPD before and after the guidelines were published and circulated to every

---

Definition of COPD

- COPD is a chronic, slowly progressive disorder characterised by airflow obstruction (reduced FEV_1 and FEV_1/VC ratio), which does not change markedly over several months

- Most of the lung function impairment is fixed, although some reversibility can be produced by bronchodilator (or other) therapy

---

Figure 12.1 Diagnosis of COPD

practice in the UK (Rudolf 1999). Pre-publication, only one third of GPs could select spirometry from a list of six tests as the test of choice for COPD. After receiving copies the figure rose to nearly half of GPs, but this would imply that fewer than that are likely actually to be ordering spirometry in their patients. In hospital the situation is not much better. A survey of 1,400 patients from 40 hospitals, all admitted with acute exacerbations of COPD (Roberts *et al.* 2001), asked if the diagnosis had been confirmed objectively. Since it was quite possible that the test would not have been done during the acute admission the survey accepted any spirometric record within the preceding five years or the three months after the index admission as acceptable. Just 51 per cent of patients had a record – 71 per cent of patients who had been managed by respiratory specialists, 49 per cent who had been looked after by non-respiratory physicians and only 27 per cent who had been under geriatricians. Yet these patients had been diagnosed and managed as COPD sufferers. Since patients with COPD are likely to be on treatment for many years, it is not unreasonable for them to expect objective confirmation that their therapy is justified.

In the patients who did have spirometry done, the results make interesting reading since there are clearly problems in interpretation. Table 12.1 shows that, while the patients under geriatricians were indeed a little older the mean lung function was similar regardless of the type of unit to which the patient had been admitted. However, the worrying feature is the range of lung function that was recorded. Patients with a forced expiratory volume in 1 second (FEV_1) of 3.5 litres and age of 70 years are essentially in the normal range and do not have COPD – and overall, approximately 5 per cent of the cohort had values over 80 per cent of predicted when those values were available. Thus, even when the data are available, there are a significant number of patients who are being wrongly labelled and thus wrongly treated, which is at best a waste of money and at worst denying them treatment for whatever condition they did have.

Table 12.1 Mean age and levels of lung function for patients admitted under the care of chest, general and geriatrician physicians

	Chest	General	Geriatric
Age (years)	71.0	70.0	75.2
FEV$_1$ levels (l)			
Mean	0.94	0.97	0.89
Median	0.80	0.88	0.73
Range	0.2–3.5	0.4–3.0	0.3–2.8

While everyone recognises the substantial overlap between asthma and COPD, in fact many of the problems of diagnosis concern other conditions. A patient aged in their 70s admitted with fluid retention may have severe COPD, i.e., cor pulmonale or may have severe ischaemic heart disease with congestive cardiac failure. Figure 12.1 illustrates how the symptoms and signs may overlap and, while it is possible that the chest radiograph may give a clue from the size of the heart, it is nothing like as good a discriminator as is the spirometric tracing. Cor pulmonale due to COPD does not occur without a severely abnormal FEV$_1$. Clearly it matters when it comes to treatment which would concentrate on low-flow oxygen in the former and on perhaps an ACE inhibitor in the latter.

Over the course of two clinics last year, the author came across three instances in which failure to measure lung function and to evaluate that information critically led to inappropriate management which in one case had continued for many years.

'The first man was referred because he wanted to be considered for early retirement on the grounds of his "emphysema" which had been treated with nebulised bronchodilators for the preceding 15 years. His occupational health physician was concerned because his FEV$_1$ was 79 per cent of predicted. I agreed that this man had no respiratory limitation and that his nebuliser was entirely inappropriate. The patient was pleased that he did not have severe emphysema but was concerned as to whether he could claim back the 15 years of prescription charges that he had paid out!'

'The second patient was referred to the clinic as COPD with an FEV$_1$ of 60 per cent of predicted that had been unresponsive to inhalers or oral steroids over some months. The FVC which was also reduced to 60 per cent of predicted had been overlooked. The eventual diagnosis was a fibrosing alveolitis possibly related to her mild rheumatoid disease.'

'The third man was 67 and had been a heavy smoker (45 pack-years) and was referred as COPD that was responding poorly and should be assessed for a nebuliser prescription. His FEV₁ was reduced (0.7 l) and on a single dose of nebuliser in the clinic it rose to 1.3 l. Later on a trial of oral steroids his FEV₁ rose to 2.7 l – his asthma, although symptomatic for many years, had never been recognised. He was delighted with the total transformation of his life.'

Accurate diagnosis does matter. Objective measurement (i.e., spirometry) is available in every hospital and many primary care practices, yet it is not routinely used.

Symptom interpretation

COPD develops from normal health through to severe respiratory incapacity as a gradually progressive disorder. The disease can only become severe having passed through mild and moderate stages first. This is important to recognise since each patient with severe disease represents a lost opportunity. If they had been discovered earlier then they might have avoided the severe stage had they been able to stop smoking. The various guidelines define mild, moderate and severe stages using different levels of FEV_1 to make the distinction but these differences are of little practical import. What does matter is that as a patient loses more lung function then symptoms are expected to increase and in large studies that is certainly true. However, when assessing individuals the situation is rather different. The relationship between FEV_1 and a patient's activity level is weak because a person's functional ability depends on more than just lung function – mood, depression, other co-morbidities all play a part. In the audit data for the 720 patients in whom both FEV_1 and performance score were recorded, the relationship between decline in function and worsening performance was present but the scatter of lung function at any one level of performance score was marked. (Figure 12.2). Performance score in this case was based on the WHO definitions used usually for cancer assessment in which a score of 1 represents normality and 5 represents a patient largely confined to the house/bed. There are patients with an FEV_1 of less than one litre who claim to be functioning normally and others with an FEV_1 of approaching two litres who claim to be almost bedridden – clearly other factors are at play but it demonstrates how difficult it can be to assess the problems in these patients.

There are no standardised assessments for COPD that can be used in routine busy clinics, although there are projects in progress that are trying to develop such tools. There are relatively long and complex quality of life scores (better called health status scores) but these are of little value in routine clinics because they take too long to record.

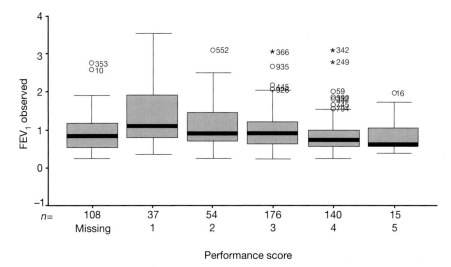

Figure 12.2 Relationship of FEV_1 with performance score in patients admitted with an acute COPD exacerbation

Selecting treatment

The guidelines suggest that more β agonists and anticholinergics be used as the severity of the COPD becomes worse. However, the outcome test that justifies continued prescription is an improvement in symptoms. Thus the profession desperately needs some reliable measures of symptoms with which to make such decisions.

Inhaled steroids are prescribed according either to a steroid reversibility test (as was recommended in the UK guidelines), whether the patient has moderate/severe disease and frequent admissions (if one accepts the ISOLDE trial – Burge *et al.* 2000), or just because the primary care physician is mixing up COPD with asthma. None of these would appear to actually be used in practice with any degree of consistency. Two thirds of acute COPD patients admitted to hospital with an exacerbation were on inhaled steroids regardless of their lung function (Roberts *et al.* 2001) and a primary care study has also noted similar findings (Peperell *et al.* 1997). In the absence of clear measures of success, prescribing in COPD will remain somewhat haphazard.

One last observation from the audit of acute exacerbations was the high numbers on oral steroids and on oral theophyllines neither of which is recommended for regular use by the UK guidelines. Old habits are slow to change.

Assessing for nebulised therapy

An example of the problems of prescribing is demonstrated by the widespread use of nebulised bronchodilators. European guidelines on the use of nebulised therapy are about to be published (O'Driscoll *et al.* 2000) and will set out guidance on the assessment of patients for nebulised therapy. In essence only patients with severe

COPD should be considered and in such patients every effort should be made to optimise existing therapy first and to ensure, for example, that the patient is able to use their usual inhalers correctly. If, after assessing all other options, the physician still wishes to prescribe a nebuliser then a trial is recommended over two or more weeks with formal monitoring of the outcome and only those with clear benefit should be continued on what is still an expensive therapeutic option. Few clinicans are as objective or systematic as is suggested by these guidelines.

A recent survey of patients on nebulised therapy attending hospitals in a UK city (Smith & Eavis 1999) showed that just over half were on nebulised treatment because of a diagnosis of COPD. However, over 40 per cent had had no objective measure of lung function recorded in their notes and those with a measure over 40 per cent did not have a severe FEV_1 deficit. In other words, the prescription of nebulisers in over half of the patients was potentially inappropriate. If the costs of treating such patients with nebulised rather than conventional inhalers is calculated, then the savings are likely to be sufficient to set up and run a COPD rehabilitation service in that city. As the ERS guidelines on nebulisers will point out, there is good evidence that rehabilitation improves the quality of life in COPD while no such evidence exists for nebulised bronchodilators.

Omissions: treatment on admission

In the same audit already referred to, data were collected as to the therapy given to the patient and in particular the use of ventilatory support (including both intermittent positive pressure ventilation [IPPV] and NIV). Only 4 per cent of patients received any form of ventilatory support. Respiratory physicians were more than twice as likely to utilise such support for their patients as non-respiratory specialists but, perhaps more remarkable, was the observation that half of the hospitals in the service did not supply ventilatory support to a single patient during the study. This is unlikely to be simply due to milder cases since in those with arterial blood gas measurements and with both acidosis (pH < 7.26) and hypercapnia only 15 per cent, i.e., less than one in six, were offered support. Most respiratory physicians would be concerned that this represents a serious level of undertreatment although one must be cautious in drawing such conclusions from a retrospective study.

Conclusions

The understanding of COPD by many UK doctors is still weak. Despite all the guidelines from all the various countries agreeing on the need for objective spirometry to make the diagnosis, the majority of patients do not have this done. The measurement and assessement of symptoms in a semi-objective manner is difficult because the tools have still not been developed and much treatment is somewhat haphazard – measures of success or not are sorely needed. In acute potentially life-threatening exacerbations, effective treatments such as the use of NIV remains patchy and suboptimal.

The 'errors' described in this chapter are a combination of a lack of knowledge about the conditon and a lack of application of what we do know. The latter can and should be tackled but the former will depend on answers emerging from new studies. The good news is the burgeoning research effort in COPD which does provide real hope for the future.

References

British Thoracic Society (1997). Guidelines for the management of chronic obstructive pulmonary disease. *Thorax* **52**, S1–28

Burge PS, Calverley PMA, Jones PW *et al.* (2000). Randomised double blind placebo-controlled trial of fluticasone propionate in patients with moderate to severe chronic obstructive pulmonary disease. *British Medical Journal* **320**, 1297–1303

O'Driscoll R, Pearson MG, Muers M (2001). Nebulisers in severe COPD. *European Respiratory Review* **10**, 516–522

Pearson MG, Littler J, Davies PDO (1994). An analysis of medical workload by speciality and diagnosis in Mersey – evidence of patient to specialist mismatch. *Journal of the Royal College of Physicians* **28**, 230–234

Peperell K, Rudolf M, Pearson MG, Diggle J (1997). General practitioner prescribing habits in asthma/COPD. *Asthma in General Practice* **5**, 29–30

Roberts CM, Ryland I, Lowe D, Kelly Y, Bucknall CE, Pearson MG (2001). Audit of acute admissions of chronic obstructive pulmonary disease – standards of care and management in the hospital setting. *European Respiratory Journal* in press

Rudolf M, on behalf of the COPD Consortium (1999). Making spirometry happen. *Thorax* **54**, A43

Smith C, Eavis JE (1999). Survey and nebulizer use across a city. *Thorax* **54**, A42

Auditing the standard of a COPD service: appraisal, accreditation and monitoring

Christine E Bucknall, C Mike Roberts and Mike G Pearson

Introduction

Chronic obstructive pulmonary disease (COPD) is a common condition and a frequent cause of acute hospital admissions, forming about half of the 25 per cent of acutely admitted patients who have respiratory disease (Pearson *et al.* 1994). Until recently it has probably also been a 'cinderella' diagnosis with an associated degree of therapeutic nihilism. It is now recognised that much can be usefully done for patients with COPD as has been shown by recent work demonstrating the benefits of pulmonary rehabilitation, non-invasive ventilation and use of long-acting β_2 agonists. These are in addition to the well-documented benefits of stopping smoking and of long-term oxygen therapy. The publication of national guidelines (British Thoracic Society 1997) has also probably played a part in the resurgence of interest in this condition and the huge expansion of research manifested by multiple sessions on COPD at national and international meetings over the last five years.

COPD audit findings

Work on COPD audit has not often been published (Angus *et al.* 1994; Neill *et al.* 1994; Tuuponen *et al.* 1997) but has shown deficiencies of care. The British Thoracic Society (BTS) audit subcommittee set out to perform a national audit in 1997 after the publication of guidelines. Volunteer hospitals collected data on 40 consecutive COPD admissions from 1 September 1997. Fourteen hundred cases were documented in this way in 38 UK hospitals (Roberts *et al.* in 2001). Wide variations in care were seen (Table 13.1) both between hospitals and between the type of physicians within a hospital. Patients discharged from the care of respiratory physicians were significantly more likely than patients of non-respiratory physicians to have received care as recommended in the national guidelines. Important aspects of care addressed in the audit included:

- had the forced expiratory volume in 1 second (FEV_1) been recorded at any time within the previous five years, i.e., had the diagnosis been objectively confirmed;
- were peak flows recorded during the admission (to assess peak expiratory flow variability and possible asthmatic component);

Table 13.1 Variability of COPD care (from Roberts *et al.* 2001)

Oxygen saturation recorded	5–100%
Blood gases measured	40–100%
Comment on chest x-ray	0–98%
Smoking advice to current smokers	0–80%
Pulmonary function tests within 5 years	0–93%
Oxygen prescribed	9–94%
Rehabilitation considered	0–39%
Mortality rate	0–50%
Readmissions	5–65%

- had inhaler technique been assessed – these elderly patients are often even less able to use inhalers correctly than younger asthma patients;
- had smoking cessation advice been given to current smokers;
- was the need for long-term oxygen therapy considered.

Variability of care and implications for standard setting

The wide variability in care is serious and cannot be written off as a benign phenomenon relating to poor note keeping, partly for medicolegal reasons where no record equates with care not delivered, and also because frequent changes in medical staff mean that good written notes are central to a good process of care. Furthermore, the study showed wide variability in outcomes, of apparently consecutive series of patients, as well as in the process of care – mortality rates varying from 0 to 50 per cent and readmissions from 5 to 65 per cent. There may be other reasons, such as differences in case mix, socio-economic factors or service availability, to explain these differences in outcome, but there is growing recognition of the utility of audit of process of care, where the process measures are robust and significant items (Mant *et al.* 1995).

A similar phenomenon was observed about ten years ago when the BTS first became involved in national audit of adults admitted to hospital with acute asthma (Pearson *et al.* 1996). Repeat audit of adult asthma care in hospital has shown improvements in care, particularly for aspects such as self-management planning where performance was generally poor originally (Bucknall *et al.* 2000). The variability of the results from individual hospitals has also diminished (unpublished data).

This raises the issue of the significance of a finding in an individual hospital. In essence, the significance of an observation as a marker of poor process of care increases as the variability of results for different hospitals diminishes, since the umbrella of normality of the bell shape enclosing the mean and 2 standard deviations becomes more tightly defined. This allows a clinically meaningful target to be set, e.g., that inhaler technique should be assessed in a minimum of 70 per cent of eligible patients, whereas, at an earlier stage in the audit process, when the variability of results was greater, the target might have to be set at 40 per cent in order to include the lower 2 standard deviations, a target that would be so low as to be useless. When this situation of minor variability of results has been achieved, standards of care with clinically meaningful targets can be set confidently, firm in the knowledge that only 1 in 20 results outside the lower 2 standard deviation bracket will be there by chance rather than because of poor process of care.

Over a number of years with repeat data a greater degree of confidence can be attached to the data and, for adult hospital asthma care, we are close to being able to set standards of care with robust and meaningful targets as described here. We also have a development plan for the COPD dataset, including validation of methods for collecting audit data on complete cohorts of patients and the reliability of data collection. This will allow ongoing audit of hospital COPD care with the aim of setting standards and targets for this condition too. The pilot data set is shown in Table 13.2.

Table 13.2 Pilot COPD audit data set

Performance status	Oral corticosteroids
Admission gases; repeat	FEV_1 within 5 years
Presence of oedema	Screening for LTOT
Comment on chest x-ray	Smoking advice
Oxygen prescribed	Inhaler technique
Ventilatory support	Letter to GP

Interpreting benchmarking data

Such audit datasets and national audit databases providing benchmarking data for comparative audit are a relative innovation in health-related quality improvement exercises in the UK and it is relevant to ask what can reasonably be expected of them, particularly in an environment where re-accreditation and revalidation of medical specialists is being actively discussed. Systems, such as that described for asthma and under development for COPD, and other respiratory topics can allow objective comment to be made on the quality of service available in an individual hospital and can therefore feed into departmental audit programmes, such as the BTS peer review scheme (Page *et al.* 1995). Together, such initiatives could allow comment to be made on the standard of specific services. They can also indirectly allow comment on the leadership of clinical services, since this is important in driving the process of change.

Even first rate leadership will not, however, remove deficiencies in care due to poor and unsupported infrastructure or inferior team working. Hospitals have probably been slow to recognise the extent to which they depend on good teamworking to function well. This operates at a number of different levels, across a range of interests:

- within medicine – consultants, middle graders and junior house staff;
- across professional groups – doctors, ward nurses, physiotherapists, respiratory nurse specialists, health service managers;
- interdepartmental – wards, radiology, laboratories.

Poor performance, as judged by the proportion of patients in a cohort having a positive comment (e.g., inhaler technique checking), will often reveal problems in teamworking and note sharing. For this reason, these systems will never provide data on individual performance, precisely because of the contribution made by a number of staff to good quality care for patients. They will therefore not be tools for revalidation in terms of providing data on performance of individuals, although they may contribute by providing documentation of involvement in quality initiatives.

What can national benchmarking contribute?

- Comment on service standards ✔

- Feed into departmental audit or appraisal systems ✔

- Provide data on individual performance ✗

- Contribute directly to revalidation ✗

Summary

Experience of the use of audit data, for COPD and other important clinical topics, is developing and there is a growing recognition of the importance of review of complete cohorts of patients, of valid and reliable data collection and of the utility of comparative audit. Systems based on these principles will have great value and can make positive contributions to quality improvement initiatives. There are limits to what can be expected of them and recognising these will also be important as their use becomes more widespread

References

Angus RM, Murray S, Kay JW, Thomson NC, Patel KR (1994). Management of chronic airflow obstruction: differences in practice between respiratory and general physicians. *Respiratory Medicine* **88**, 493–497

British Thoracic Society (1997). Guidelines for the management of chronic obstructive pulmonary disease. *Thorax* **52**, S1–28

Bucknall CE, Ryland I, Cooper A, Coutts II, Connolly CK, Pearson MG (2000). National benchmarking as a support system for clinical governance. *Journal of the Royal College of Physicians* **34**, 52–56

Mant J & Hicks N (1995). Detecting differences in quality of care: how sensitive are process and outcome measures in the treatment of acute myocardial infarction? *British Medical Journal* **311**, 793–796

Neill AM, Epton MJ, Martin IR, Drennan CJ, Town GI (1994). An audit of the assessment and management of patients admitted to Christchurch Hospital with chronic obstructive airways disease. *New Zealand Medical Journal* **107**, 365–367

Page RL & Harrison BDW (1995). Setting up interdepartmental peer review. *Journal of the Royal College of Physicians* **29**, 319–324

Pearson MG, Littler J, Davies PDO (1994). An analysis of medical workload by specialty and diagnosis in Mersey: evidence of a specialist to patient mismatch. *Journal of the Royal College of Physicians* **28**, 230–234

Pearson MG, Ryland I, Harrison BDW (1996). Comparison of the process of care of acute severe asthma in adults admitted to hospital before and 1 year after the publication of guidelines. *Respiratory Medicine* **90**, 539–545

Roberts CM, Ryland I, Lowe D, Kelly Y, Bucknall CE, Pearson MG (2001). Audit of acute admissions with COPD – standards of care and management in the hospital setting *European Respiratory Journal* in press

Tuuponen T, Keistinen T, Kivela S (1997). Regional differences in long term mortality among hospital treated asthma and COPD patients. *Scandinavian Journal of the Society of Medicine* **25**, 238–242

Index